Pharmacologic

CLASSIFICATION OF DRUGS

with Doses and Preparations

FIFTH EDITION

KD Tripathi MD
Ex-Director-Professor and Head of Pharmacology
Maulana Azad Medical College and associated
LN and GB Pant Hospitals, New Delhi

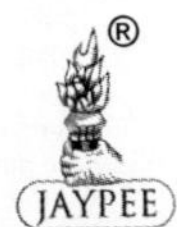

JAYPEE BROTHERS MEDICAL PUBLISHERS (P) LTD

New Delhi • London • Philadelphia • Panama

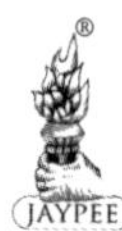

Jaypee Brothers Medical Publishers (P) Ltd

Headquarters

Jaypee Brothers Medical Publishers (P) Ltd
4838/24, Ansari Road, Daryaganj
New Delhi 110 002, India
Phone: +91-11-43574357
Fax: +91-11-43574314
Email: jaypee@jaypeebrothers.com

Overseas Offices

J.P. Medical Ltd
83, Victoria Street, London
SW1H 0HW (UK)
Phone: +44-2031708910
Fax: +02-03-0086180
Email: info@jpmedpub.com

Jaypee-Highlights Medical Publishers Inc.
City of Knowledge, Bld. 237, Clayton
Panama City, Panama
Phone: +1 507-301-0496
Fax: +1 507-301-0499
Email: cservice@jphmedical.com

Jaypee Medical Inc
The Bourse
111 South Independence Mall East
Suite 835, Philadelphia, PA 19106, USA
Phone: +1 267-519-9789
Email: joe.rusko@jaypeebrothers.com

Jaypee Brothers Medical Publishers (P) Ltd
17/1-B Babar Road, Block-B, Shaymali
Mohammadpur, Dhaka-1207
Bangladesh
Mobile: +08801912003485
Email: jaypeedhaka@gmail.com

Jaypee Brothers Medical Publishers (P) Ltd
Bhotahity, Kathmandu, Nepal
Phone: +977-9741283608
Email: kathmandu@jaypeebrothers.com

Website: www.jaypeebrothers.com
Website: www.jaypeedigital.com

Inquiries for bulk sales may be solicited at: jaypee@jaypeebrothers.com

Pharmacological Classification of Drugs with Doses and Preparations

First Edition: 1986, Second Edition: 1990, Third Edition: 2006, Fourth Edition: 2010, *Fifth Edition*: **2014**

ISBN 978-93-5152-108-2

Printed at Sanat Printers, Kundli

Pharmacological

CLASSIFICATION OF DRUGS

with Doses and Preparations

Preface

A systematized listing of drugs according to their primary actions, mechanisms, chemical nature, clinical uses and/or other relevant characteristics is the first step to learn about them. The mental exercise to prescribe a drug for a patient starts with identifying the class of drugs to be prescribed and then selecting the specific member most appropriate for that patient according to its subclass/group/individual characteristic. For example, the first thing one decides is whether an analgesic or an antihypertensive or an antibiotic is to be prescribed; then proceeds to consider which type of analgesic (opioid/nonopioid), or antihypertensive (β blocker/ACE inhibitor, etc.), or antibiotic (β-lactam/fluoroquinolone, etc.) is required and then which specific member is most suitable. On the other hand, every drug is known by its class and subclass, e.g. furosemide is a high-ceiling diuretic, glibenclamide is a sulfonylurea antidiabetic. As such, drug classifications are pivotal to pharmacology students and highly valuable to prescribing doctors. The phenomenal increase in the number of drugs in recent years has further underscored the need for drug classifications.

Drug classifications have been criticised for being arbitrary and imperfect because of nonuniform criteria that have often to be adopted and frequent lack of watertight distinctions among drug groups/subgroups. Nevertheless, basing on pharmacological differences and applying practical criteria, meaningful drug classifications can be devised. Though, any drug has multiple actions/properties, it can be designated by the most outstanding one. For example, labelling atenolol as a cardioselective β blocker summarises its actions, uses, etc. This booklet has adopted such a pragmatic approach and presented classifications of drugs that have been well accepted. The outstanding feature of the present edition is reformating of the classifications in the form of eye-catching charts. These charts create pictorial images and help memorizing. All classifications have been updated, modified where necessary and newer drugs have been included, particularly those marketed recently.

To be useful to medical/pharmacy students as well as to practitioners, the doses (including pediatric doses wherever relevant), frequency and route(s) of administration along with leading brand names of drugs and different types of dosage forms (oral, parenteral, topical, etc.) are listed distinctively after each class of drugs. Thus, essential prescribing information is incorporated for drugs that are available. Single drug formulations are mainly mentioned. Combined drug formulations find a place wherever important or relevant. The listing of brand names is restricted to only 1–4 per drug, and is not exhaustive. Synonyms and alternative names of drugs and classes of drugs are also mentioned. Two separate indices, one of nonproprietary (generic) names and the other of proprietary (brand) names of drugs is provided for instantaneous location of the drug or the product one is looking for.

It is hoped that the present user-friendly format of the booklet will make it a better aid to remembering drug names, identifying the class and subclass to which they belong, and provide easy access to core prescribing information. The credit for meticulous production of this booklet goes to the staff of M/s Jaypee Brothers.

KD Tripathi

Explanatory Notes

1. The information on dosage form(s) is printed in maroon colour, and the proprietary (brand) names of drugs/products appear in capital letters.
2. The doses and regimens are given in smaller type, while nonproprietary (generic) drug names appear in bigger type and different font.
3. If no brand name of a drug is listed, it is not currently marketed in India, or is marketed only in combinations. This can be found out from the composition of the combined formulations given.
4. If the route of administration is not specified, the drug is administered only orally, and the dose mentioned is the oral dose.
5. Drug doses mentioned without specifying frequency of administration indicate the quantity for a single dose.

Abbreviations

amp	Ampoule
AP	Action potential
BD	Twice daily
BHP	Benign hypertrophy of prostate
BSA	Body surface area
cap	Capsule
Ch	Child dose
cm	Centimeter
CR	Continuous release
Distab	Dispersible tablet
DS	Double strength
DTPA	Diethylene triamine pentaacetic acid
e.c.	Enteric coated
ER	Extended release
ERP	Effective refractory period
ext	Extract
g	Gram
GITS	Gastrointestinal therapeutic system
hr	hour
i.d.	Intradermal
i.m.	Intramuscular
inj	Injection
IU	International unit
i.v.	intravenous
kg	Kilogram
L	Litre
LES	Lower esophageal sphincter
liq	Liquid
m	Meter
max	Maximum
mEq	Milliequivalent
mg	Milligram
min	Minute
ml	Millilitre
MR	Modified release
MU	Mega (million) unit
MW	Molecular weight
μg	Microgram
OD	Once daily
oint	Ointment

Pot.	Potassium
QID	Four times a day
rDNA	Recombinant deoxyribonucleic acid
s.c.	Subcutaneous
s.l.	Sublingual
Sod	Sodium
SR	Sustained release
susp	Suspension
syr	Syrup
tab	Tablet
$TCID_{50}$	Tissue culture infective dose 50%
TDS	Three times a day
THFA	Tetrahydrofolic acid
TTS	Transdermal therapeutic system
U	Unit
UV	Ultra violet
yr	Year (age)
ZE	Zollinger-Ellison

Contents

1 Drugs Acting on Autonomic Nervous System

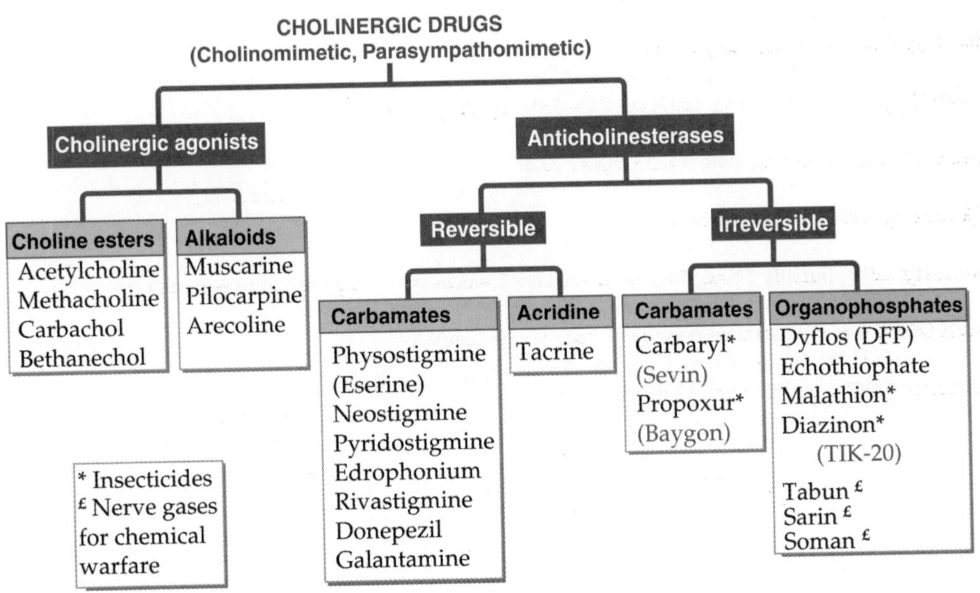

Preparations

1. **Bethanechol:** 10–40 mg oral, 2.5–5 mg s.c.
   UROTONIN, BETHACOL 25 mg tab.
2. **Pilocarpine:** 0.5–4% topically in eye.
   PILOCAR 1%, 2%, 4% eye drops; CARPINE 0.5% eye drops; PILODROPS 2% eye drops.
3. **Physostigmine:** 0.5–1.0 mg oral/i.m., 0.25–0.5% topically in eye.
   BI-MIOTIC 0.25% eye drops with 2% pilocarpine nitrate.
4. **Neostigmine:** 15–30 mg oral, 0.5–2.5 mg s.c./i.m.
   PROSTIGMIN, MYOSTIGMIN, TILSTIGMIN 15 mg tab, 0.5 mg/ml in 1 ml and 5 ml inj.
5. **Pyridostigmine:** 60–180 mg oral.
   DISTINON, MYESTIN 60 mg tab.
6. **Rivastigmine:** Initially 1.5 mg BD, increase every 2 weeks by 1.5 mg/day upto 6 mg BD.
   EXELON, RIVAMER 1.5, 3, 4.5, 6.0 mg caps.
7. **Donepezil:** 5 mg at bed time once daily (max 10 mg/day).
   DONECEPT, DOPEZIL, DORENT 5, 10 mg tabs.
8. **Galantamine:** 4 mg BD (max 12 mg BD).
   GALAMER 4, 8, 12 mg tabs.

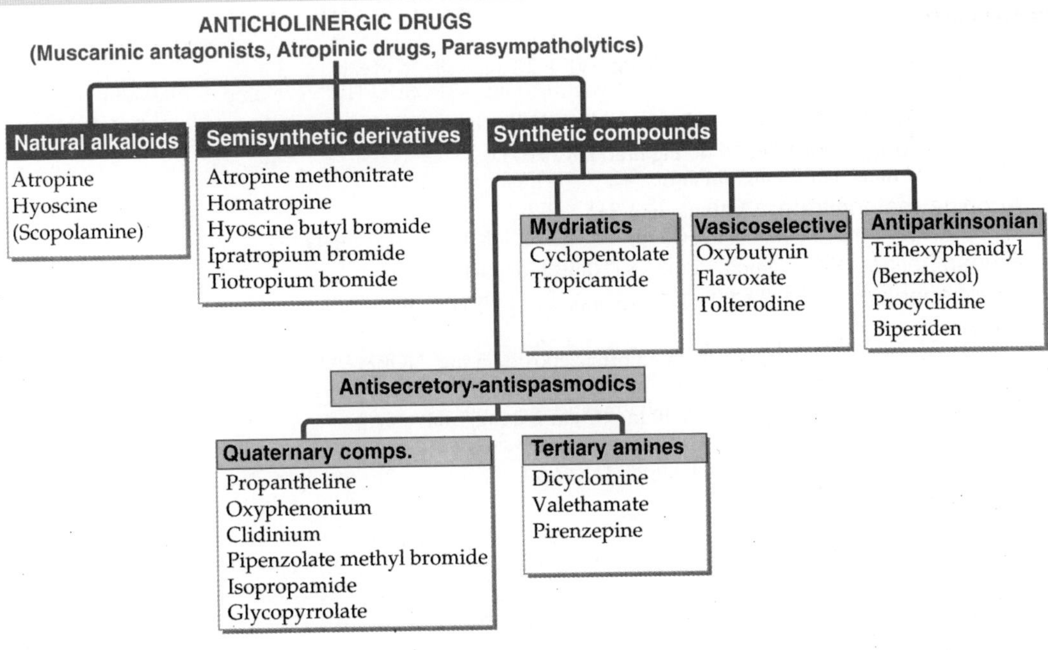
ANTICHOLINERGIC DRUGS
(Muscarinic antagonists, Atropinic drugs, Parasympatholytics)
Natural alkaloids
Atropine
Hyoscine
(Scopolamine)
Semisynthetic derivatives
Atropine methonitrate
Homatropine
Hyoscine butyl bromide
Ipratropium bromide
Tiotropium bromide
Synthetic compounds
Mydriatics
Cyclopentolate
Tropicamide
Vasicoselective
Oxybutynin
Flavoxate
Tolterodine
Antiparkinsonian
Trihexyphenidyl
(Benzhexol)
Procyclidine
Biperiden
Antisecretory-antispasmodics
Quaternary comps.
Propantheline
Oxyphenonium
Clidinium
Pipenzolate methyl bromide
Isopropamide
Glycopyrrolate
Tertiary amines
Dicyclomine
Valethamate
Pirenzepine

Preparations

1. **Atropine:** 0.6–2.0 mg i.m./i.v. (Child 10 μg/kg), 1–2% topically in eye.
   ATROPINE SULPHATE 0.6 mg/ml inj, 1% eye drop/oint, ATROSULPH 1% eye drop, 5% eye oint.
2. **Hyoscine hydrobromide:** 0.3–0.5 mg oral/i.m. (Child 10 μg/kg).
3. **Hyoscine butyl bromide:** 20–40 mg oral/i.m./s.c./i.v.
   BUSCOPAN 10 mg tab, 20 mg/ml amp.
4. **Atropine methonitrate:** 2.5–10 mg oral/i.m.
   MYDRINDON 1 mg (adult), 0.1 mg (child) tab; in SPASMOLYSIN 0.32 mg tab.
5. **Propantheline:** 15–30 mg oral. PROBANTHINE 15 mg tab.
6. **Oxyphenonium:** 5–10 mg (Child 3–5 mg) oral. ANTRENYL 5, 10 mg tab.
7. **Clidinium:** 2.5–5 mg oral.
   In SPASRIL, ARWIN 2.5 mg tab with chlordiazepoxide 5 mg. NORMAXIN, CIBIS 2.5 mg with dicyclomine 10 mg and chlordiazepoxide 5 mg tab.
8. **Pipenzolate methyl bromide:** 5–10 mg (Child 2–3 mg) oral.
   In PIPEN 5 mg tab. 4 mg/ml drops with dimethyl polysiloxane.
9. **Isopropamide:** 5 mg oral. In STELABID, GASTABID 5 mg tab. with trifluoperazine.
10. **Dicyclomine:** 20 mg oral.
    CYCLOSPAS-D 20 mg with dimethicone 40 mg tab; CYCLOPAM INJ. 10 mg/ml in 2 ml, 10 ml, 30 ml amp/vial, also 20 mg tab with paracetamol 500 mg; in COLIMEX, COLIRID 20 mg with paracetamol 500 mg tab, 10 mg/ml drops with dimethicone.
11. **Valethamate:** 8 mg i.m., 10 mg oral, repeated as required.
    VALAMATE 8 mg in 1 ml inj, EPIDOSIN 10 mg tab, 8 mg inj.

12. **Glycopyrrolate:** 0.1–0.3 mg i.m./i.v., 1–2 mg oral.
GLYCO-P 0.2 mg/ml amp., 1 mg in 5 ml vial, PYROLATE 0.2 mg/ml, 1 ml amp, 10 ml vial.
13. **Ipratropium bromide:** 40–80 μg by inhalation/nasal spray.
IPRAVENT 20 μg/puff metered dose inhaler, 2 puffs 3–4 times daily; 250 μg/ml respirator soln., 0.4–2 ml nebulized in conjunction with a β_2 agonist 2–4 times daily.
Also used to control rhinorrhoea in perennial rhinitis and common cold; IPRANASE–AQ 0.084% nasal spray (42 μg per actuation), 1–2 sprays in each nostril 3–4 times a day.
14. **Tiotropium bromide:** 18 μg by inhalation. TIOVA 18 μg rotacaps, 1 rotacap by inhalation OD.
15. **Oxybutynin:** 5 mg BD/TDS oral; children above 5 yr 2.5 mg BD.
OXYBUTIN, CYSTRAN, OXYSPAS 2.5 mg and 5 mg tabs.
16. **Flavoxate:** 200 mg TDS. URISPAS, FLAVATE, FLAVOSPAS 200 mg tab.
17. **Tolterodine:** 1–2 mg BD or 2–4 mg OD of sustained release tab. oral; ROLITEN, TOLTER 1, 2 mg tabs, TORQ 2, 4 mg SR tab.
18. **Homatropine:** 1–2% topically in eye. HOMATROPINE EYE, HOMIDE 1%, 2% eye drops.
19. **Cyclopentolate:** 0.5–1.0% topically in eye.
CYCLOMID EYE, 0.5%, 1.0%, CYCLOGYL, CYCLOPENT 1% eye drops.
20. **Tropicamide:** 0.5–1.0% topically in eye. OPTIMIDE, TROPICAMET, TROMIDE 1% eye drops; TROPAC-P, TROPICAMET PLUS 0.8% + phenylephrine 5% eye drops.
21. **Trihexyphenidyl (benzhexol):** 2–10 mg/day; PACITANE, PARBENZ 2 mg tab.
22. **Procyclidine:** 5–20 mg/day; KEMADRIN 2.5, 5 mg tab.
23. **Biperiden:** 2–10 mg/day oral, i.m. or i.v.: DYSKINON 2 mg tab., 5 mg/ml inj.

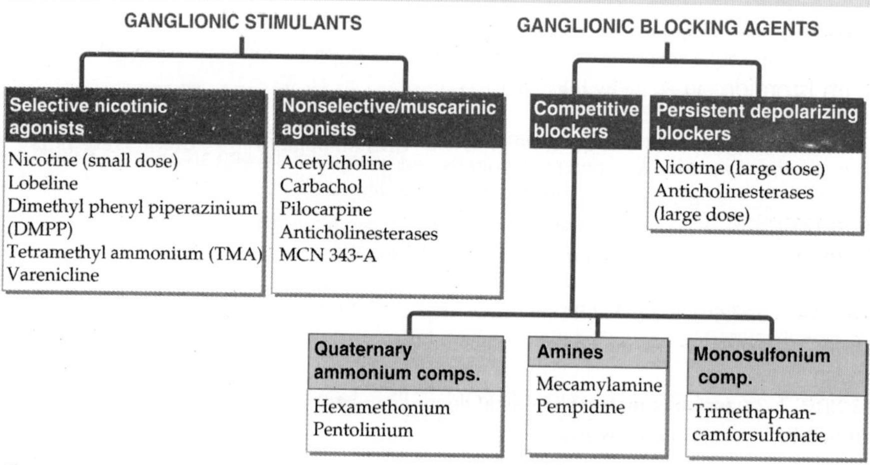

Preparations

1. **Nicotine transdermal:** NICOTINELL-TTS 10, 20, 30 cm² patches releasing 7, 14, 21 mg nicotine per 24 hr respectively. In those smoking > 20 cigarettes every day—start with 30 cm² patch, shift to smaller patches every 3–5 days, treat for 3–4 weeks.
2. **Nicotine chewing gum:** NULIFE 1, 2, 4 mg chewing gum; In those smoking > 20 cigarettes/day—start with 4 mg gum chewed slowly for 30 min when urge to smoke occurs—gradually reduce to 2 mg gum and then 1 mg gum. In less heavy smokers—start at lower doses.

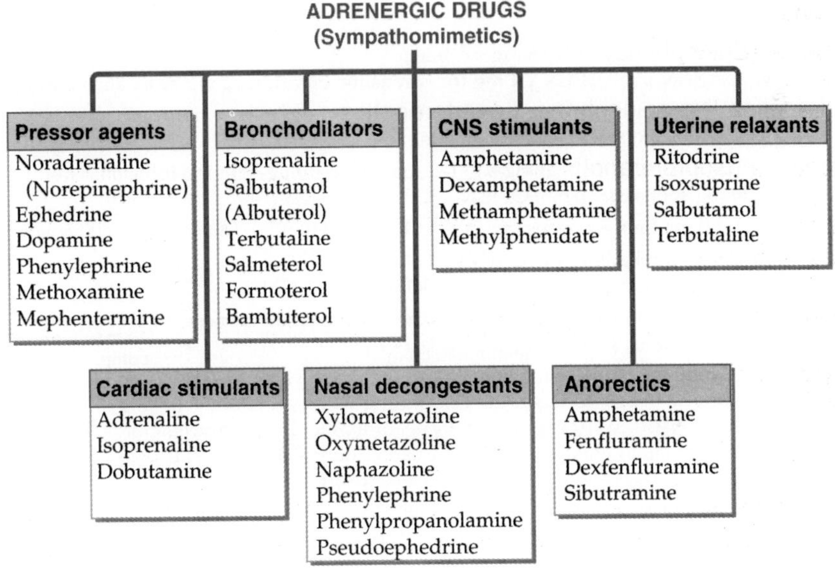
ADRENERGIC DRUGS
(Sympathomimetics)
Pressor agents
Noradrenaline
(Norepinephrine)
Ephedrine
Dopamine
Phenylephrine
Methoxamine
Mephentermine
Bronchodilators
Isoprenaline
Salbutamol
(Albuterol)
Terbutaline
Salmeterol
Formoterol
Bambuterol
CNS stimulants
Amphetamine
Dexamphetamine
Methamphetamine
Methylphenidate
Uterine relaxants
Ritodrine
Isoxsuprine
Salbutamol
Terbutaline
Cardiac stimulants
Adrenaline
Isoprenaline
Dobutamine
Nasal decongestants
Xylometazoline
Oxymetazoline
Naphazoline
Phenylephrine
Phenylpropanolamine
Pseudoephedrine
Anorectics
Amphetamine
Fenfluramine
Dexfenfluramine
Sibutramine

Preparations

1. **Adrenaline (Epinephrine):** 0.2–0.5 mg s.c./i.m.;
ADRENALINE 1 mg/ml inj; ADRENA 4 mg (of adrenaline bitartrate=2 mg adrenaline base) per ml inj.
2. **Noradrenaline (Norepinephrine, Levarterenol):** 2–4 μg/min i.v. infusion;
ADRENOR, NORAD, NORDRIN 2 mg (base)/2 ml amp.
3. **Isoprenaline (Isoproterenol):** 20 mg s.l., 1–2 mg i.m., 5–10 μg/min i.v. infusion;
NEOEPININE 20 mg sublingual tab, ISOPRIN, ISOSOL 4 mg/2 ml inj.
4. **Dopamine:** 0.2–1.0 mg/min i.v. infusion; DOPAMINE, INTROPIN, DOPACARD 200 mg/5 ml amp.
5. **Dobutamine:** 2.5–10 μg/kg/min i.v. infusion;
CARDIJECT 50 mg/4 ml and 250 mg/20 ml inj, DOBUTREX, DOBUSTAT 250 mg inj.
6. **Ephedrine:** 15–60 mg oral, 15–30 mg i.m./i.v.; 0.5–0.75% topically in nose. EPHEDRINE HCL 15, 30 mg tabs, SUFIDRIN 50 mg in 1 ml inj, ENDRINE 0.75% nasal drops.
7. **Phenylephrine:** 5–10 mg oral, 2–5 mg i.m., 0.1–0.5 mg slow i.v. inj, 30–60 μg/min i.v. infusion, 0.25% topically in nose, 5–10% topically in eye; in DECOLD PLUS 5 mg with paracetamol 400 mg + chlorpheniramine 2 mg + caffeine 15 mg tab; SINAREST 10 mg with chlorpheniramine 2 mg, paracetamol 500 mg, caffeine 30 mg tab; FRENIN 10 mg in 1 ml inj, in FENOX 0.25% with naphazoline 0.025% nasal drops, DROSYN 10% eye drops, in DROSYN-T, TROPAC-P 5% with tropicamide 0.8% eye drops.
8. **Methoxamine:** 10–20 mg i.m., 3–5 mg slow i.v. inj; VASOXINE 20 mg/ml inj.
9. **Mephentermine:** 10–20 mg oral/i.m., also by i.v. infusion.
MEPHENTINE 10 mg tab, 15 mg in 1 ml amp, 30 mg/ml in 10 ml vial.
10. **Amphetamine:** 5–15 mg oral.
11. **Dexamphetamine:** 5–10 mg (children 2.5–5 mg) oral.
12. **Methamphetamine:** 5–10 mg oral.

13. **Sibutramine:** Start with 10 mg OD, increase to 15 mg OD if needed.
14. **Xylometazoline:** 0.05%–0.1% topically in nose;
    OTRIVIN 0.05% (pediatric), 0.1% (adult) nasal drops and nasal spray.
15. **Oxymetazoline:** 0.025–0.05% topically in nose;
    NASIVION, SINAREST 0.025% (pediatric), 0.05% (adult) nasal drops.
16. **Naphazoline:** 0.1% topically in nose; PRIVINE 0.1% nasal drops.
17. **Pseudoephedrine:** 30–60 mg oral TDS; SUDAFED 60 mg tab, 30 mg/5 ml syrup; in SINAREST 60 mg with chlorpheniramine 2 mg + caffeine 30 mg + paracetamol 500 mg tab; in CHESTON 30 mg with chlorpheniramine 2 mg + bromhexine 4 mg per tab and per 5 ml syr; in ACTICOLD 60 mg with chlorpheniramine 4 mg + paracetamol 500 mg tab; in CODYLEX 60 mg with chlorpheniramine 4 mg + ibuprofen 400 mg tab.
18. **Phenylpropanolamine:** 25–50 mg TDS; In ACTIFED 25 mg with triprolidine 2.5 mg tab; in ESKOLD 50 mg with diphenylpyraline 5 mg spansule; in FLUCOLD 25 mg with chlorpheniramine 2 mg + paracetamol 500 mg tab.
19. **Ritodrine:** 50–200 μg/min i.v. infusion, 10 mg i.m./oral 4–6 hourly; YUTOPAR, RITROD 10 mg/ml inj (5 ml amp), 10 mg tab. RITODINE 10 mg tab, 10 mg in 1 ml inj.
20. **Isoxsuprine:** 5–10 mg oral, i.m. 4–6 hourly, DUVADILAN 10 mg tab, 40 mg SR cap, 10 mg/2 ml inj.

Note: For doses and preparations of β_2 agonist bronchodilators (salbutamol, etc.) *See* p. 34.

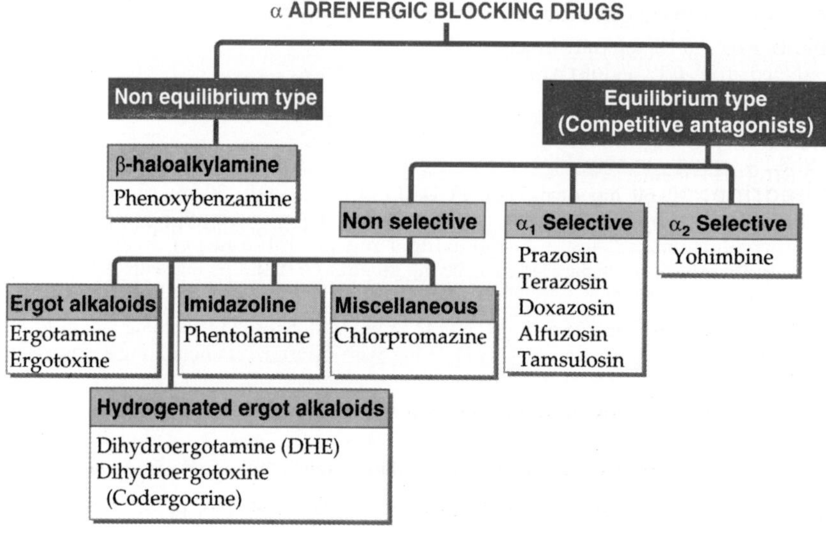
α ADRENERGIC BLOCKING DRUGS
Non equilibrium type
β-haloalkylamine
Phenoxybenzamine
Equilibrium type (Competitive antagonists)
Non selective
Ergot alkaloids
Ergotamine
Ergotoxine
Imidazoline
Phentolamine
Miscellaneous
Chlorpromazine
Hydrogenated ergot alkaloids
Dihydroergotamine (DHE)
Dihydroergotoxine (Codergocrine)
α1 Selective
Prazosin
Terazosin
Doxazosin
Alfuzosin
Tamsulosin
α2 Selective
Yohimbine

Preparations

1. **Phenoxybenzamine:** 20–60 mg/day oral, 1 mg/kg slow i.v. infusion over 1 hour; FENOXENE 10 mg cap, 50 mg/ml inj, BIOPHENOX 50 mg/ml inj.
2. **Ergotamine:** For migraine 1–3 mg oral/sublingual, repeat as required (max 6 mg in a day); rarely 0.25–0.5 mg i.m. or s.c.; ERGOTAMINE, GYNERGEN, INGAGEN 1 mg tab, 0.5 mg/ml and 1 mg/ml inj.
3. **Dihydroergotamine:** For migraine 2–6 mg oral (max 10 mg/day), 0.5–1 mg i.m., s.c. repeat hourly (max 3 mg); DIHYDERGOT, DHE 1 mg tab, MIGRANIL 1 mg/ml inj.
4. **Dihydroergotoxine (codergocrine):** For dementia 1–1.5 mg oral or sublingual, 0.15–0.6 mg i.m., HYDERGINE 1.5 mg tab, CERELOID 1 mg tab.
5. **Phentolamine:** 5 mg i.v. repeated as required; REGITINE, FENTANOR 10 mg/ml inj.
6. **Prazosin:** Start with 0.5–1 mg at bedtime; usual dose 1–4 mg BD or TDS; PRAZOPRES 0.5, 1.0 and 2.0 mg tabs. MINIPRESS XL: PRAZOSIN GITS 2.5 mg and 5 mg tablets; 1 tab OD.
7. **Terazosin:** Usual maintenance dose 2–10 mg OD; HYTRIN, TERALFA, OLYSTER 1, 2, 5 mg tab.
8. **Doxazosin:** 1 mg OD initially, increase upto 8 mg BD; DOXACARD, DURACARD, DOXAPRESS 1, 2, 4 mg tabs.
9. **Alfuzosin:** 2.5 BD-QID or 10 mg OD as modified release tab. ALFUSIN, ALFOO 10 mg ER tab.
10. **Tamsulosin:** URIMAX, DYNAPRES 0.2, 0.4 mg MR cap; CONTIFLO-OD 0.4 mg cap; 1 cap (max 2) in the morning with meals.
11. **Yohimbine:** 2 mg oral; YOHIMBINE 2 mg tab.

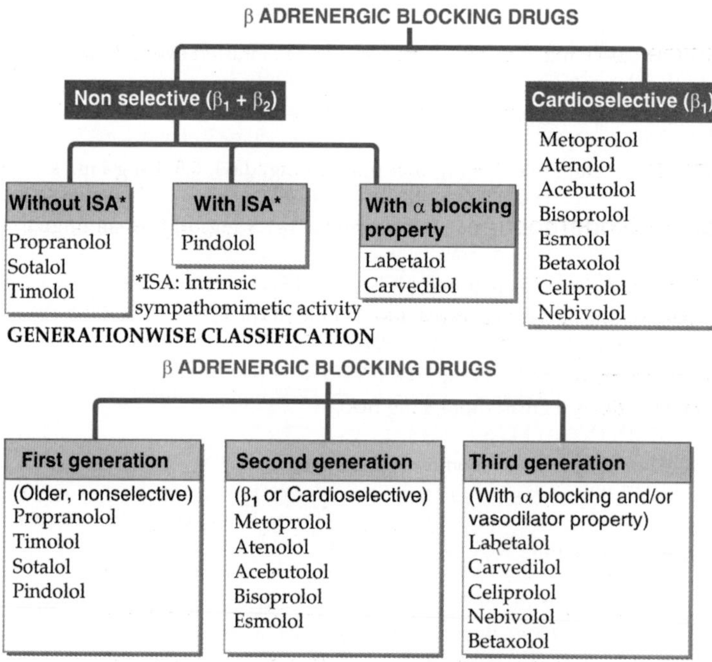
β ADRENERGIC BLOCKING DRUGS
Non selective ($\beta_1 + \beta_2$)
Cardioselective (β_1)
Metoprolol
Atenolol
Acebutolol
Bisoprolol
Esmolol
Betaxolol
Celiprolol
Nebivolol
Without ISA*
Propranolol
Sotalol
Timolol
With ISA*
Pindolol
With α blocking property
Labetalol
Carvedilol
*ISA: Intrinsic sympathomimetic activity
GENERATIONWISE CLASSIFICATION
β ADRENERGIC BLOCKING DRUGS
First generation
(Older, nonselective)
Propranolol
Timolol
Sotalol
Pindolol
Second generation
(β_1 or Cardioselective)
Metoprolol
Atenolol
Acebutolol
Bisoprolol
Esmolol
Third generation
(With α blocking and/or vasodilator property)
Labetalol
Carvedilol
Celiprolol
Nebivolol
Betaxolol

Preparations

1. **Propranolol:** Oral—10 mg BD to 160 mg QID (average 40–160 mg/day). Start with a low dose and gradually increase according to need; i.v.—2 to 5 mg injected over 10 min with constant monitoring. It is not injected s.c. or i.m. because of irritant property. INDERAL, CIPLAR 10, 40, 80 mg tab, 1 mg/ml inj., BETABLOC 10, 40 mg tab.
2. **Sotalol:** 80 mg BD–160 mg TDS oral; SOTAGARD 40, 80 mg tabs.
3. **Pindolol:** 5–15 mg BD; PINADOL 5 mg tab, VISKEN 10, 15 mg tab.
4. **Metoprolol:** 25 mg BD–100 mg QID oral, 5–15 mg slow i.v. inj;
   BETALOC 25, 50, 100 mg tab, 5 mg/ml inj., LOPRESOR, METOLAR 50, 100 mg tab.
5. **S(–) Metoprolol:** 12.5 mg BD–50 mg QID; METPURE-XL 12.5, 25, 50 mg ER tabs.
6. **Atenolol:** 25 mg OD–50 mg BD; BETACARD, ATEN, TENORMIN 25, 50, 100 mg tabs.
7. **S(–) Atenolol:** 12.5–50 mg OD; ATPURE, ADBETA 12.5, 25, 50 mg tabs.
8. **Acebutolol:** 200 mg BD–400 mg TDS oral; 20–40 mg slow i.v. injection; SECTRAL 200, 400 mg tabs, 10 mg/2 ml amp.
9. **Bisoprolol:** 2.5–10 mg OD; CONCOR, CORBIS 5 mg tab.
10. **Esmolol:** 0.5 mg/kg i.v. injection followed by 0.05–0.2 mg/kg/min i.v. infusion;
    MINIBLOCK 100 mg/10 ml, 250 mg/10 ml inj.
11. **Celiprolol:** 100 mg OD–300 mg BD; CELIPRES 100, 200 mg tab.
12. **Nebivolol:** 5 mg OD (start with 2.5 mg OD in elderly); NODON 5 mg tab, NEBICARD 2.5, 5 mg tabs.
13. **Labetalol:** Start with 50 mg BD, increase to 100–200 mg TDS oral. In hypertensive emergencies 20–40 mg slow i.v. injection every 10 min till desired response is obtained.
    NORMADATE 50, 100, 200 mg tab; LABESOL, LABETA 50 mg tab, 20 mg/4 ml inj.
14. **Carvedilol:** *for CHF:* Start with 3.125 mg BD for 2 weeks, if well tolerated, gradually increase to max. of 25 mg BD.
    for hypertension/angina: 6.25 mg BD initially, titrate to max. of 25 mg BD.
    CARVIL, CARLOC, CARVAS 3.125, 6.25, 12.5, 25 mg tabs; ORICAR 12.5, 25 mg tabs.

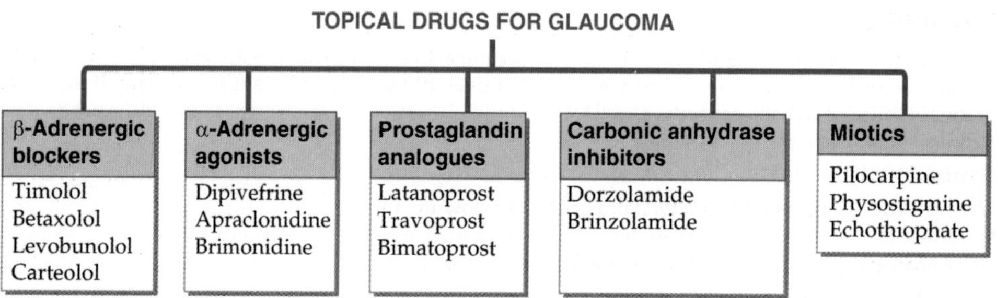

Preparations

1. **Timolol:** Start with 0.25% eye drops BD, change to 0.5% drops in case of inadequate response. 0.5% OD as gel forming solution. GLUCOMOL, OCUPRES, IOTIM, LOPRES 0.25% and 0.5% eye drops. TIMOLAST 0.5% gel forming eye drops (long acting).

   Timolol 0.5% + Latanoprost 0.005%: LAPROST PLUS, LATOCHEK-T eye drops.
2. **Betaxolol:** 0.5% topically in eye BD; OPTIPRES, IOBET, OCUBETA 0.5% eye drops.
3. **Levobunolol:** 0.5% topically in eye OD; BETAGAN 0.5% ophthalmic solution.
4. **Dipivefrine:** 0.1% topically in eye BD; PROPINE 0.1% eye drops.
5. **Apraclonidine:** 0.5–1.0% topically in eye; ALFADROPS-DS 1% eye drops.
6. **Brimonidine:** 0.2% topically in eye TDS;
   ALPHAGAN-P, BRIMODIN-P 0.15% eye drops, IOBRIM 0.2% eye drops.

7. **Latanoprost:** 0.005% topically in eye OD in evening; LACOMA, XALATAN, LATOPROST, 9 PM 50 μg/ml eye drops; LACOMA-T, LAPROST-PLUS, LATOCHEK-T with timolol 0.5% eye drops (store in cold place).
8. **Travoprost:** 0.004% topically in eye OD in evening; TRAVATAN 0.004% eye drops (refrigeration of the eye drops not required); TRAVACOM 0.004% with timolol 0.5% eye drops.
9. **Bimatoprost:** 0.03% as eye drops OD in evening; LUMIGAN, CAREPROST 0.03% eye drops; the eye drop need not be stored in refrigerator; CAREPROST-PLUS, GANFORT with timolol 0.5% eye drop.
10. **Pilocarpine:** 0.5%–4% topically in eye; CARPINE, PILOCAR 0.5%, 1%, 2%, 4% eye drops.
11. **Dorzolamide:** 2% topically in eye BD–TDS; DORTAS, DORZOX 2% eye drops.

2 Autacoids and Related Drugs

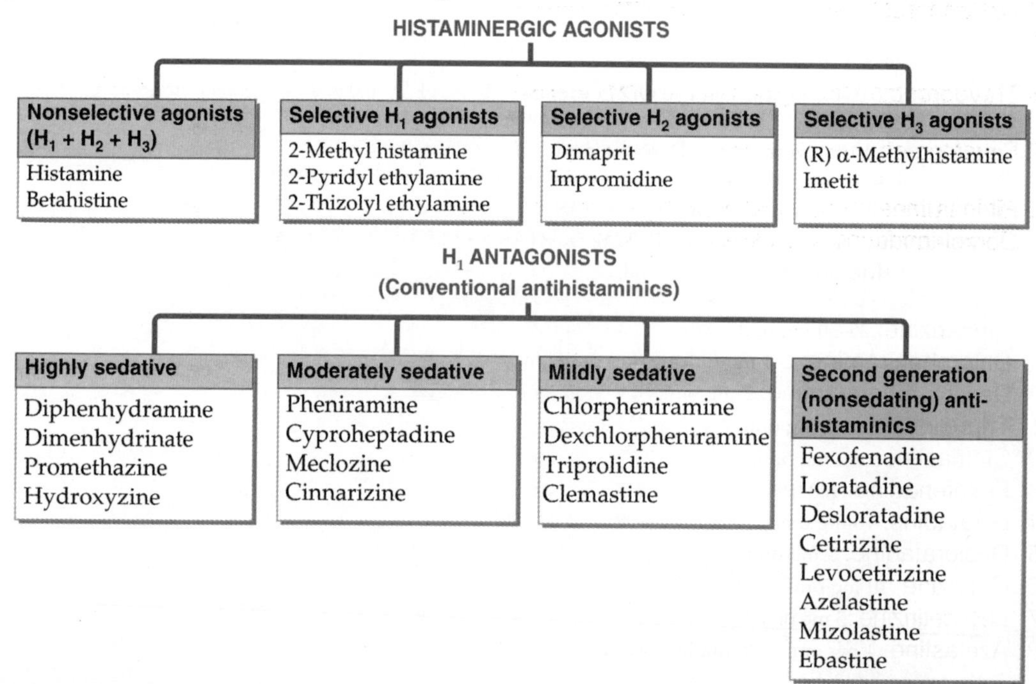

Preparations

Betahistine (Histaminergic agonist): 4–8 mg 6–8 hourly; VERTIN 8 mg tab.

1. Diphenhydramine: 25–50 mg oral; BENADRYL 25 mg cap, 12.5 mg/5 ml syr.
2. Dimenhydrinate: 25–50 mg oral, i.m.; DRAMAMINE 16 mg/5 ml syr, 50 mg tab, GRAVOL 50 mg tab.
3. Promethazine: 25–50 mg oral, i.m. (1 mg/kg); PHENERGAN 10, 25 mg tab., 5 mg/ml elixer, 25 mg/ml inj.
4. Hydroxyzine: 25–50 mg oral, i.m.; ATARAX 10, 25 mg tab., 10 mg/5 ml syr, 6 mg/ml drops, 25 mg/ml inj.
5. Pheniramine: 20–50 mg oral, i.m.; AVIL 25 mg, 50 mg tab, 15 mg/5 ml syr, 22.5 mg/ml inj.
6. Cyproheptadine: 4 mg oral; PRACTIN, CIPLACTIN 4 mg tab., 2 mg/5 ml syrup.
7. Meclozine (Meclizine): 25–50 mg oral;
   In DILIGAN 12.5 mg + niacin 50 mg tab., In PREGNIDOXIN 25 mg + Caffeine 20 mg tab.
8. Cinnarizine: 25–50 mg oral; STUGERON, VERTIGON 25 and 75 mg tab.
9. Chlorpheniramine: 2–4 mg (0.1 mg/kg) oral, i.m.; PIRITON, CADISTIN 4 mg tab.
10. Dexchlorpheniramine: 2 mg oral; POLARAMINE 2 mg tab., 0.5 mg/5 ml syrup.
11. Triprolidine: 2.5–5 mg oral; ACTIDIL 2.5 mg tab, ACTIFED 2.5 mg with pseudoephedrine 60 mg.
12. Clemastine: 1–2 mg oral; TAVEGYL 1 mg tab., 0.5 mg/5 ml syr.
13. Fexofenadine: 120–180 mg oral; ALLEGRA, ALTIVA, FEXO 120, 180 mg tab.
14. Loratadine: 10 mg oral; LORFAST, LORIDIN, LORMEG, 10 mg tab, 1 mg/ml susp.
15. Desloratadine: 5 mg oral; DESLOR, LORDAY, NEOLORIDIN 5 mg tab.
16. Cetirizine: 10 mg oral; ALERID, CETZINE, ZIRTIN, SIZON 10 mg tab, 5 mg/5 ml syr.
17. Levocetirizine: 5 mg oral; LEVORID, LEVOSIZ 5 mg, 10 mg tab, TECZINE, LEVOCET 5 mg tab, 2.5 mg/5 ml syr.
18. Azelastine: 4 mg oral, 0.28 mg intranasal; AZEP NASAL SPRAY 0.14 mg per puff nasal spray.

19. **Mizolastine:** 10 mg oral; ELINA 10 mg tab.
20. **Ebastine:** 10 mg oral; EBAST 10 mg tab.
21. **Rupatadine:** 10 mg oral; RUPAHIST 10 mg tab.

Note: For H_2-Antagonists (H_2-Antihistaminics) *See* p. 118, 119.

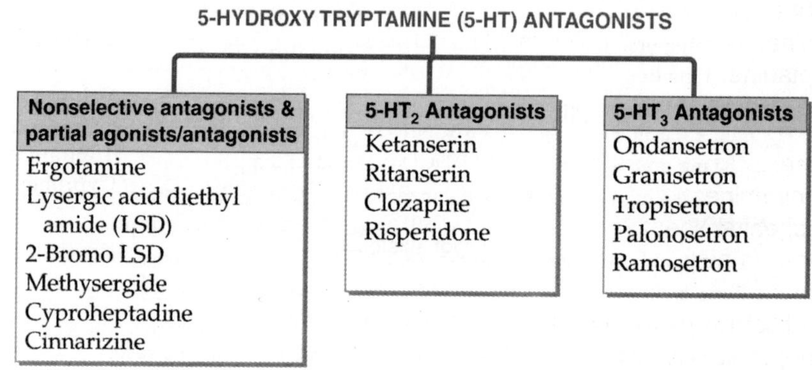

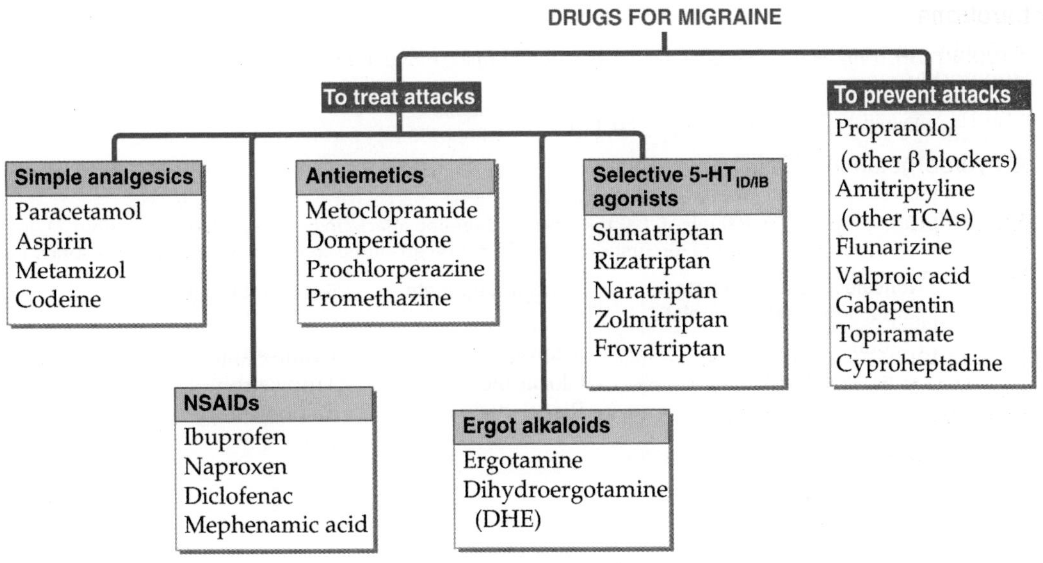
DRUGS FOR MIGRAINE
To treat attacks
To prevent attacks
Simple analgesics
Paracetamol
Aspirin
Metamizol
Codeine
Antiemetics
Metoclopramide
Domperidone
Prochlorperazine
Promethazine
Selective 5-HT ID/IB agonists
Sumatriptan
Rizatriptan
Naratriptan
Zolmitriptan
Frovatriptan
Propranolol
(other β blockers)
Amitriptyline
(other TCAs)
Flunarizine
Valproic acid
Gabapentin
Topiramate
Cyproheptadine
NSAIDs
Ibuprofen
Naproxen
Diclofenac
Mephenamic acid
Ergot alkaloids
Ergotamine
Dihydroergotamine
(DHE)

Preparations

1. **Ergotamine:** 1 mg oral/sublingual, repeat as required (max. 6 mg), 0.25–0.5 mg s.c./i.m.;
   ERGOTAMINE 1 mg tab, 0.5 mg/ml inj.
   MIGRIL: Ergotamine 2 mg, caffeine 100 mg, cyclizine 50 mg tab.
   VASOGRAIN: Ergotamine 1 mg, caffeine 100 mg, paracetamol 250 mg, prochlorperazine 2.5 mg tab.
2. **Dihydroergotamine (DHE):** 2–6 mg oral (max. 10 mg/day), 0.5–1.0 mg i.m., s.c.; DHE 1 mg tab, MIGRANIL 1 mg/ml inj.
3. **Sumatriptan:** 6 mg s.c., 50–100 mg oral at the onset of migraine attack, may be repeated once within 24 hours if required. Those not responding to the first dose should not be given the second dose; 25 mg nasal spray, may be repeated once after 2 hours;
   SUMINAT, SUMITREX 25, 50, 100 mg tabs, MIGRATAN 50, 100 mg tabs, SUMITREX-INJ KIT 6 mg in 0.5 ml inj.; also SUMINAT 25 mg per actuation nasal spray.
4. **Rizatriptan:** 5-10 mg at the onset of migraine attack, may be repeated after 2 hours if required.Those not responding to the first dose should not be given the second dose; RIZACT, RIZATAN 5 mg, 10 mg tabs.
5. **Flunarizine:** 10–20 mg OD, children 5 mg OD; NOMIGRAIN, FLUNARIN 5 mg, 10 mg caps/tab.

Note: For preparations of other drugs, *see* Index.

PROSTAGLANDINS (PGs)

Natural PGs	Prostaglandin analogues
Dinoprostone (PGE_2)	Carboprost (15-methyl $PGF_{2\alpha}$)
Gemeprost	Misoprostol (methyl PGE_1 ester)
Dinoprost ($PGF_{2\alpha}$)	Latanoprost (PGE_2 analogue)
Alprostadil (PGE_1)	Travoprost
Prostacyclin (PGI_2) (Epoprostenol)	Bimatoprost

Prostaglandins (PGs)

1. **PGE_2 (Dinoprostone):** PROSTIN-E_2 for induction/augmentation of labour, midterm abortion.
   Vaginal gel (1 mg or 2 mg in 2.5 ml) 1 mg inserted into posterior fornix, followed by 1–2 mg after 6 hour if required.
   Vaginal tab (3 mg) 3 mg inserted into posterior fornix, followed by another 3 mg if labour does not start within 6 hour.
   Extraamniotic solution (10 mg/ml in 0.5 ml amp.) infrequently used.
   Intravenous solution (1 mg/ml in 0.75 ml amp., 10 mg/ml in 0.5 ml amp) i.v. route rarely used, more side effects.
   Oral tablet PRIMIPROST 0.5 mg tab, one tab. hourly till induction, max 1.5 mg per hr; rarely used.
   Cervical gel CERVIPRIME (0.5 mg in 2.5 ml prefilled syringe) 0.5 mg inserted into cervical canal for preinduction cervical softening and dilatation in patients with poor Bishop's score.
2. **Gemeprost:** CERVAGEM 1 mg vaginal pessary: for softening of cervix in first trimester–1 mg 3 hr before attempting dilatation; for 2nd trimester abortion/molar gestation—1 mg every 3 hours, max. 5 doses.
3. **$PGF_{2\alpha}$ (Dinoprost):** PROSTIN F_2 ALPHA intraamniotic injection, 5 mg/ml in 4 ml amp. for midterm abortion/induction of labour (rarely used).
4. **15-methyl $PGF_{2\alpha}$ (Carboprost):** PROSTODIN 0.25 mg in 1 ml amp; 0.25 mg i.m. every 30–120 min for PPH, midterm abortion, missed abortion.
5. **Misoprostol (methyl–PGE_1 ester):** 200 μg oral 6 hourly; CYTOLOG 200 μg tab, MISOPROST 100, 200 μg tab. T-PILL + MISO Mifepristone 200 mg tab (3 tabs) + misoprostol 200 μg (2 tabs); mifepristone 3 tab orally followed 2 days later by misoprostol 2 tab orally for termination of pregnancy of upto 49 days.
6. **PGE_1 (Alprostadil):** 0.5 mg by slow i.v. infusion; PROSTIN–VR, BIOGLANDIN 0.5 mg in 1 ml inj.
7. **PGI_2 (Prostacyclin, Epoprostenol):** 0.5 mg by i.v. infusion or injection in extracorporeal circulation; |FLOLAN 0.5 mg per vial for reconstitution.

Note: For preparations of other analogues, *see* Index.

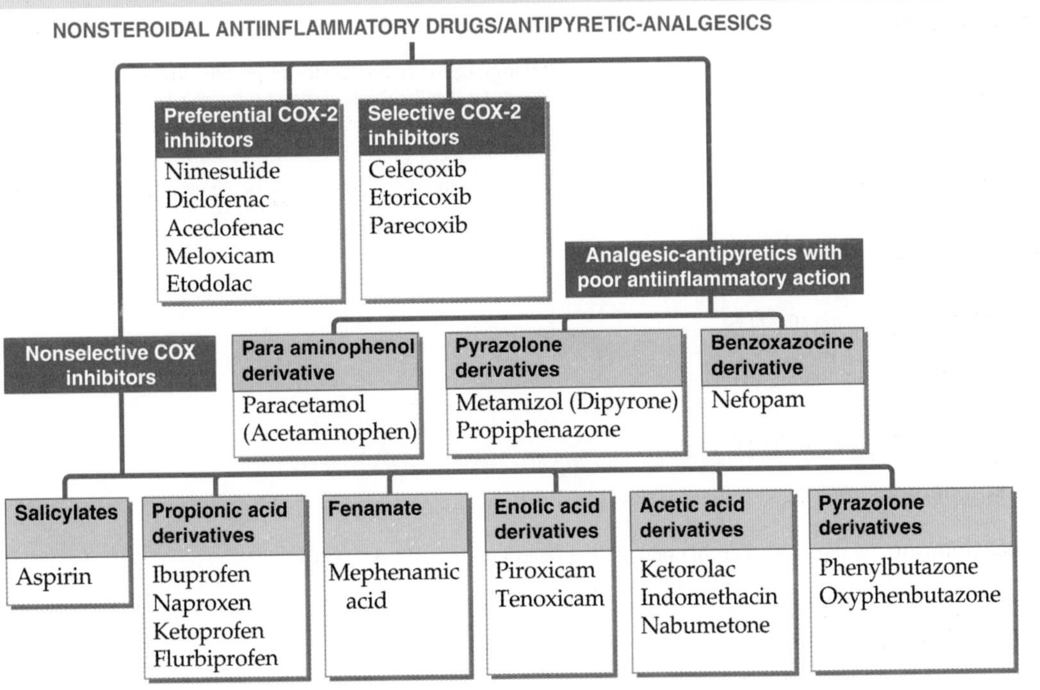
NONSTEROIDAL ANTIINFLAMMATORY DRUGS/ANTIPYRETIC-ANALGESICS
Preferential COX-2 inhibitors
Nimesulide
Diclofenac
Aceclofenac
Meloxicam
Etodolac
Selective COX-2 inhibitors
Celecoxib
Etoricoxib
Parecoxib
Analgesic-antipyretics with poor antiinflammatory action
Para aminophenol derivative
Paracetamol (Acetaminophen)
Pyrazolone derivatives
Metamizol (Dipyrone)
Propiphenazone
Benzoxazocine derivative
Nefopam
Nonselective COX inhibitors
Salicylates
Aspirin
Propionic acid derivatives
Ibuprofen
Naproxen
Ketoprofen
Flurbiprofen
Fenamate
Mephenamic acid
Enolic acid derivatives
Piroxicam
Tenoxicam
Acetic acid derivatives
Ketorolac
Indomethacin
Nabumetone
Pyrazolone derivatives
Phenylbutazone
Oxyphenbutazone

Preparations

1. **Aspirin:** Antiinflammatory dose 3–5 g/day (75–100 mg/kg/day); analgesic-antipyretic dose 0.3–0.6 g 6–8 hourly; antiplatelet dose 75–150 mg/day. ASPIRIN 350 mg tab, COLSPRIN 100, 325 mg tabs, ECOSPRIN 75, 150, 325 mg tabs, DISPRIN 325 mg (with calcium carbonate 105 mg + citric acid 35 mg) tab, LOPRIN 75, 162.5 mg tabs.

   BIOSPIRIN: Lysine acetylsalicylate 900 mg + glycine 100 mg/vial for dissolving in 5 ml water and i.v. injection.
2. **Indomethacin:** 25–50 mg BD–QID. Those not tolerating the drug orally may be given nightly suppository. IDICIN, INDOCAP 25 mg cap, 75 mg SR cap, ARTICID 25, 50 mg cap, INDOFLAM 25, 75 mg caps, 1% eye drop. RECTICIN 50 mg suppository.
3. **Ibuprofen:** 400–800 mg TDS;
   BRUFEN, EMFLAM, IBUSYNTH 200, 400, 600 mg tab, IBUGESIC also 100 mg/5 ml susp.
4. **Naproxen:** 250 mg BD–TDS;
   NAPROSYN, NAXID, ARTAGEN, XENOBID 250 mg tab, NAPROSYN also 500 mg tab.
5. **Ketoprofen:** 50–100 mg BD–TDS;
   KETOFEN 50, 100 mg tab; OSTOFEN 50 mg cap. RHOFENID 100 mg tab, 200 mg SR tab; 100 mg/2 ml amp.
6. **Flurbiprofen:** 50 mg BD–QID;
   ARFLUR 50, 100 mg tab, 200 mg SR tab, FLUROFEN 100 mg tab, OCUFLUR 0.03% eye drops.
7. **Mephenamic acid:** 250–500 mg TDS; MEDOL 250, 500 mg cap; MEFTAL 250, 500 mg tab, 100 mg/5 ml susp. PONSTAN 125, 250, 500 mg tab, 50 mg/ml syrup.
8. **Diclofenac:** 50 mg TDS, then BD oral, 75 mg deep i.m.; VOVERAN, DICLONAC, MOVONAC 50 mg enteric coated tab, 100 mg S.R. tab, 25 mg/ml in 3 ml amp. for i.m. inj. DICLOMAX 25, 50 mg tab, 75 mg/3 ml inj.

   Diclofenac potassium: VOLTAFLAM 25, 50 mg tab, ULTRA-K 50 mg tab; VOVERAN 1% topical gel.
9. **Aceclofenac:** 100 mg BD; ACECLO, DOLOKIND 100 mg tab, 200 mg SR tab.

10. **Piroxicam:** 20 mg BD for two days followed by 20 mg OD; DOLONEX, PIROX 10, 20 mg cap, 20 mg dispersible tab, 20 mg/ml inj in 1 and 2 ml amps; PIRICAM 10, 20 mg cap.
11. **Tenoxicam:** 20 mg OD; TOBITIL 20 mg tab.
12. **Ketorolac:** 10–20 mg oral 6 hourly, 15–30 mg i.m./i.v. 6 hourly (max 90 mg/day); KETOROL, ZOROVON, KETANOV, TOROLAC 10 mg tab, 30 mg in 1 ml amp., KETLUR, ACULAR 0.5% eye drops.
13. **Nimesulide:** 100 mg BD; NIMULID, NIMEGESIC, NIMODOL 100 mg tab, 50 mg/5 ml susp.
14. **Meloxicam:** 7.5–15 mg OD; MELFLAM, MEL–OD, MUVIK, M–CAM 7.5 mg, 15 mg tabs.
15. **Nabumetone:** 500 mg OD; NABUFLAM 500 mg tab.
16. **Etodolac:** 200-400 mg BD-TDS; ETOVA 200, 300, 400 mg tabs.
17. **Celecoxib:** 100–200 mg BD; CELACT, CELCOX, COLCIBRA, COBIX 100, 200 mg tabs.
18. **Etoricoxib:** 60–120 mg OD; TOROCOXIA, ETOXIB, ETOSHINE, NUCOXIA 60, 90, 120 mg tabs.
19. **Parecoxib:** 40 mg oral/i.m./i.v. repeated after 6–12 hours (max. 80 mg/day); PAROXIB 40 mg tab, REVALDO, VALTO-P 40 mg/vial inj.
20. **Paracetamol:** 325–650 mg (children 10–15 mg/kg) 3-5 times a day (max. 2600 mg/day); also 80–250 mg as suppository in infants and children; CROCIN 0.5 g tab, 125 mg/5 ml and 250 mg/5 ml syr, 100 mg/ml pediatric drops, CROCIN PAIN RELIEF 650 mg with caffeine 50 mg tab; METACIN, PARACIN 500 mg tab, 125 mg/5 ml syrup, 150 mg/ml ped. drops, ULTRAGIN, PYRIGESIC, CALPOL 500 mg tab, 125 mg/5 ml syrup, NEOMOL, FEVASTIN, FEBRINIL 300 mg/2 ml inj. JUNIMOL-RDS 80, 170, 250 mg suppository, PARACETAMOL RECTAL SUPPOSITORY 80, 170 mg.
21. **Metamizol:** 0.5–1.5 g oral/i.m./i.v.; ANALGIN 0.5 g tab; NOVALGIN, BARALGAN 0.5 g tab, 0.5 g/ml in 2 ml and 5 ml amps; ULTRAGIN 0.5 g/ml inj in 2 ml amp and 30 ml vial.

22. **Propiphenazone:** 300–600 mg TDS; marketed only in combination in several 'over the counter' preparations–in SARIDON, ANAFEBRIN: propiphenazone 150 mg + paracetamol 250 mg tab, DART: propiphenazone 150 mg + paracetamol 300 mg + caffeine 50 mg tab.
23. **Nefopam:** 30–60 mg TDS oral, 20 mg i.m. 6 hourly; NEFOMAX 30 mg tab, 20 mg in 1 ml amp.

Topical NSAIDs

1. **Diclofenac 1% gel:** VOLINI GEL, RELAXYL GEL, DICLONAC GEL
2. **Ibuprofen 10% gel:** RIBUFEN GEL
3. **Naproxen 10% gel:** NAPROSYN GEL
4. **Ketoprofen 2.5% gel:** RHOFENID GEL
5. **Flurbiprofen 5% gel:** FROBEN GEL
6. **Nimesulide 1% gel:** NIMULID TRANS GEL, ZOLANDIN GEL, NIMEGESIC-T-GEL
7. **Piroxicam 0.5% gel:** DOLONEX GEL, MOVON GEL, PIROX GEL, MINICAM GEL

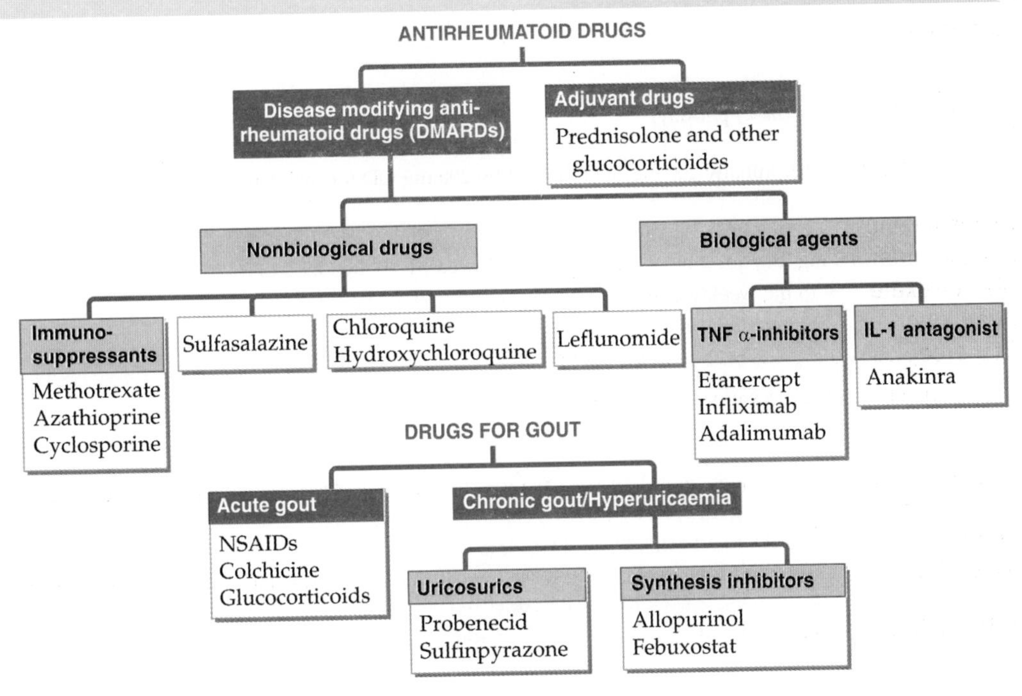
ANTIRHEUMATOID DRUGS
Disease modifying anti-rheumatoid drugs (DMARDs)
Adjuvant drugs
Prednisolone and other glucocorticoides
Nonbiological drugs
Biological agents
Immuno-suppressants
Methotrexate
Azathioprine
Cyclosporine
Sulfasalazine
Chloroquine
Hydroxychloroquine
Leflunomide
TNF α-inhibitors
Etanercept
Infliximab
Adalimumab
IL-1 antagonist
Anakinra
DRUGS FOR GOUT
Acute gout
NSAIDs
Colchicine
Glucocorticoids
Chronic gout/Hyperuricaemia
Uricosurics
Probenecid
Sulfinpyrazone
Synthesis inhibitors
Allopurinol
Febuxostat

Preparations

Antirheumatoid drugs

1. **Chloroquine:** 150 mg (base) per day;
   LARIAGO, RESOCHIN, NIVAQUIN-P 250 mg as phosphate (150 mg base) tab.
2. **Hydroxychloroquine:** initially 200 mg BD followed by 200 mg OD for maintenance;
   ZHQUINE, ZYQ 200 mg tab.
3. **Sulfasalazine:** 1–3 g/day in 2–3 divided doses; SALAZOPYRIN, SAZO-EN 0.5 g tab.
4. **Leflunomide:** 100 mg/day for 3 days loading dose followed by 20 mg OD; LEFRA 10 mg, 20 mg tabs.
5. **Methotrexate:** 7.5–15 mg weekly oral; NEOTREXATE, BIOTREXATE 2.5 mg tab.
6. **Azathioprine:** 50–150 mg/day; IMURAN 50 mg tab.
7. **Etanercept:** 25–50 mg s.c. once or twice weekly; ENBREL, ENBROL 25 mg/0.5 ml and 50 mg/1 ml inj.

Note: For preparations of corticosteroids, *see* Index.

Drugs for gout

1. **Colchicine:** For control of acute attack – 0.5 mg 1–3 hourly to a total of 3 doses; maintenance dose 0.5–1 mg/day; for prophylaxis 0.5–1.5 mg/day; ZYCOLCHIN, GOUTNIL 0.5 mg tab.
2. **Probenecid:** 0.25–1.0 g BD; BENEMID, BENCID 0.5 g tab.
3. **Allopurinol:** Start with 100 mg OD, gradually increase to maintenance dose of 300 mg/day; maximum 600 mg/day. ZYLORIC 100, 300 mg tabs., ZYLOPRIM, CIPLORIC 100 mg cap.
4. **Febuxostat:** 40–80 mg OD; FABULAS, FABUSTAT, ZURIG, 40, 80, 120 mg tabs.

3 Drugs for Respiratory Disorders

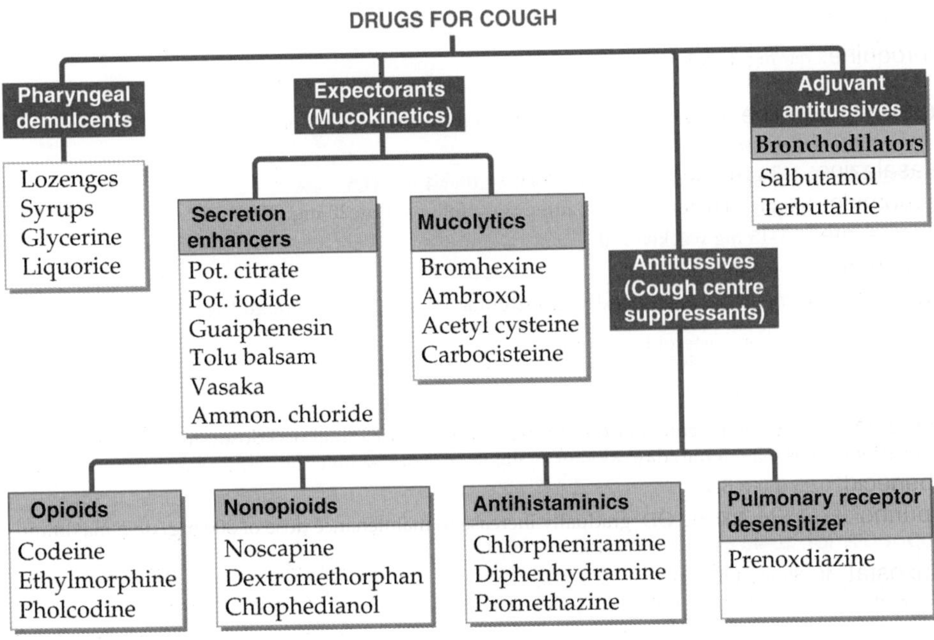

Preparations

1. **Sod./Pot. citrate/acetate:** 0.3–1.0 g TDS.
2. **Guaiphenesin:** 100–200 mg TDS.
3. **Tolu balsam:** 0.3–0.6 g TDS.
4. **Vasaka syrup:** 2–4 ml TDS.
5. **Ammonium chloride:** 50–200 mg TDS.
6. **Bromhexine:** 8 mg TDS, child 1–5 yr 4 mg BD, 5–10 yr 4 mg TDS; BROMHEXINE 8 mg tab, 4 mg/5 ml elixer.
7. **Ambroxol:** 15–30 mg TDS;
   AMBRIL, AMBROLITE, AMBRODIL, MUCOLITE 30 mg tab, 30 mg/5 ml liq, 7.5 mg/ml drops.
8. **Carbocisteine:** 250–750 mg TDS; MUCODYNE 375 mg cap, 250 mg/5 ml syr.
9. **Acetylcysteine:** 200 mg/ml solution by nebulization or instillation through tracheostomy tube;
   MUCOMIX 200 mg/ml inj in 1, 2, 5 ml amps.
10. **Codeine:** 15–30 mg TDS; children 2–6 years 7.5 mg, 6–12 years 15 mg; CODINE 15 mg tab, 15 mg/5 ml linctus.
11. **Ethylmorphine:** 10-30 mg TDS; DIONINDON 16 mg tab.
12. **Pholcodine:** 10–15 mg BD–TDS.
13. **Noscapine:** 15–30 mg, children 2–6 years 7.5 mg, 6–12 years 15 mg;
    COSCOPIN 7 mg/5 ml syrup, COSCOTABS 25 mg tab.
14. **Dextromethorphan:** 10–20 mg TDS, child 2–6 yr 2.5–5 mg, 6–10 yrs 5–10 mg.
15. **Chlophedianol:** 20–40 mg BD–TDS;
    DETIGON, TUSSIGON 20 mg/5 ml linctus with Ammon. chloride 50 mg and menthol 0.25 mg.
16. **Prenoxdiazine:** 100–200 mg TDS. PRENOXID 100, 200 mg tab.

Some combined antitussive-expectorant formulations

ASTHALIN EXPECTORANT: Salbutamol 2 mg, guaiphenesin 100 mg per 10 ml syr; dose 10–20 ml.

ASCORIL-C: Codeine 10 mg, chlorpheniramine 4 mg per 5 ml syr.

AXALIN: Ambroxol 15 mg, guaiphenesin 50 mg, salbutamol 1 mg, menthol 1 mg per 5 ml syr.

BRONCHOSOLVIN: Guaiphenesin 100 mg, terbutaline 2.5 mg, bromhexine 8 mg per 10 ml susp.

CADICOFF, GRILINCTUS: Dextromethorphan 5 mg, chlorpheniramine 2.5 mg, guaiphenesin 50 mg, amm. chloride 60 mg per 5 ml syr.

BENADRYL COUGH FORMULA: Diphenhydramine 14 mg, amm. chlor. 138 mg, sod. citrate 57 mg, menthol 1.1 mg per 5 ml syrup; dose 5–10 ml, children 2.5–5 ml.

BRO-ZEDEX: Bromhexine 8 mg, guaiphenesin 100 mg, terbutaline 2.5 mg, menthol 5 mg per 10 ml syrup; dose 10 ml.

CADISTIN EXPECTORANT: Chlorpheniramine 2 mg, glyceryl guaiacolate 80 mg, amm. chlor. 100 mg, sod. citrate 44 mg, menthol 0.8 mg, terpin hydrate 4 mg, tolu balsam 6 mg, vasaka syrup 0.13 ml per 5 ml syrup; dose 10 ml.

CHERICOF: Dextromethorphan 10 mg, chlorpheniramine 2 mg, phenylpropanolamine 12.5 mg per 5 ml liq.

CLISTIN: Dextromethorphan 10 mg, Carbinoxamine 4 mg, amm. chlor. 240 mg, sod. citrate 240 mg per 10 ml syrup.

COREX: Chlorpheniramine 4 mg, codeine phos. 10 mg, menthol 0.1 mg per 5 ml syrup; dose 5 ml, children 1.25–2.5 ml.

COSCOPIN LINCTUS: Noscapine 7 mg, chlorpheniramine 2 mg, citric acid 29 mg, sod. citrate 3 mg, amm. chlor. 28 mg per 5 ml syrup; dose 10–20 ml.

COSOME: Bromhexine 8 mg, phenylephrine 10 mg, chlorpheniramine 4 mg per 10 ml syr; dose 10 ml.

SOLVIN EXPECTORANT: Bromhexine 4 mg, pseudoephedrine 30 mg tablet and in 10 ml liquid; dose 1 tablet or 5 ml liquid.

TOSSEX: Codeine phos 10 mg, chlorpheniramine 4 mg, menthol 1.5 mg, sod. citrate 75 mg per 5 ml liquid; dose 5 ml.

VENTORLIN EXPECTORANT: Salbutamol 2 mg, guaiphenesin 100 mg per 10 ml syrup; dose 10 ml, children 2.5–7.5 ml.

ZEET EXPECTORANT: Diphenhydramine 8 mg, amm. chlor. 100 mg, guaiphenesin 50 mg, bromhexine 4 mg, menthol 1 mg per 5 ml syr.

ZEET LINCTUS: Dextromethorphan 10 mg, guaiphenesin 50 mg, phenylpropanolamine 25 mg per 5 ml syr; dose 5 ml.

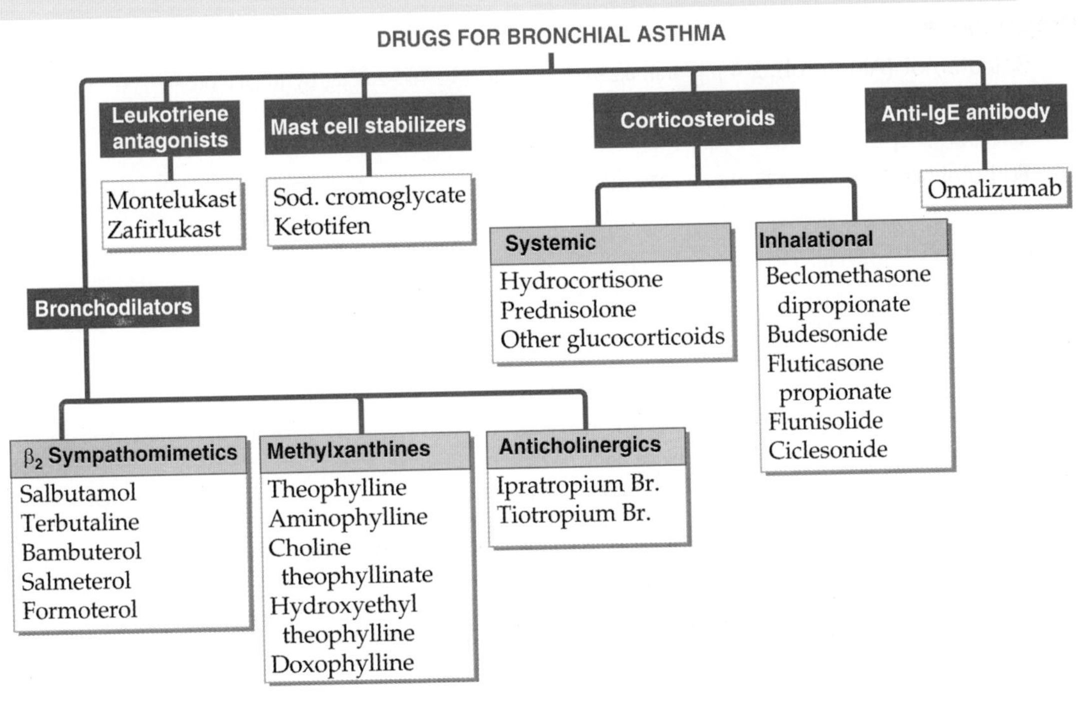
DRUGS FOR BRONCHIAL ASTHMA
Leukotriene antagonists
Montelukast
Zafirlukast
Mast cell stabilizers
Sod. cromoglycate
Ketotifen
Corticosteroids
Systemic
Hydrocortisone
Prednisolone
Other glucocorticoids
Inhalational
Beclomethasone dipropionate
Budesonide
Fluticasone propionate
Flunisolide
Ciclesonide
Anti-IgE antibody
Omalizumab
Bronchodilators
β2 Sympathomimetics
Salbutamol
Terbutaline
Bambuterol
Salmeterol
Formoterol
Methylxanthines
Theophylline
Aminophylline
Choline theophyllinate
Hydroxyethyl theophylline
Doxophylline
Anticholinergics
Ipratropium Br.
Tiotropium Br.

Preparations

1. **Salbutamol (Albuterol):** 2–4 mg oral, 0.25–0.5 mg i.m./s.c., 100–200 μg by inhalation; ASTHALIN 2, 4 mg tab., 8 mg SR tab., 2 mg/5 ml syrup, 100 μg metered dose inhaler; 5 mg/ml respirator soln., 200 μg rota caps; CROYSAL 0.5 mg/ml inj, SALOL 2.5 mg/3 ml inj; VENTORLIN 2 mg/5 ml syr, 4 mg, 8 mg CR caps., DERIHALER 100 μg metered dose inhaler.
2. **Terbutaline:** 5 mg oral, 0.25 mg s.c., 250 μg by inhalation; TERBUTALINE, BRICAREX 2.5, 5 mg tab., 3 mg/5 ml syrup, 0.5 mg/ml inj; MISTHALER 250 μg/metered dose, 10 mg/ml nebulizing soln.; BRICANYL 0.5 mg/ml inj, 2.5 mg, 5 mg tabs, 1.5 mg/5 ml syr.
3. **Bambuterol:** 10–20 mg OD in the evening;
   BAMBUDIL 10 mg, 20 mg tabs, 5 mg/5 ml oral soln; BETADAY 10, 20 mg tabs.
4. **Salmeterol:** 50–100 μg by inhalation;
   SALMETER, SEROBID 25 μg per metered dose inhaler; 2 puffs BD; severe cases 4 puffs BD; also SEROBID ROTACAPS 50 μg; 1–2 caps BD by inhalation.
   SEROFLO—100/250/500 ROTACAPS: Salmeterol 50 μg + fluticasone 100 μg/250 μg/500 μg per rotacap
   SEROFLO—125/250, COMBITIDE—125/250, INHALERS: Salmeterol 25 μg + fluticasone 125 μg or 250 μg per puff.
5. **Formoterol:** 12–24 μg by inhalation twice daily; FORATEC 12 μg rotacaps.
6. **Theophylline (anhydrous):** 100–300 mg TDS (15 mg/kg/day), THEOLONG 100, 200 mg SR cap., DURALYN-CR 400 mg continuous release cap, UNICONTIN 400 mg, 600 mg CR tabs, THEOBID 200, 300 mg tabs.
7. **Aminophylline (Theophylline-ethylenediamine; 85% theophylline):** water soluble, can be injected i.v. but not i.m. or s.c., 250–500 mg oral or slow i.v. injection; children 7.5 mg/kg i.v.; AMINOPHYLLINE 100 mg tab, 250 mg/10 ml inj.
8. **Hydroxyethyl theophylline (Etophylline, 80% theophylline):** water soluble; can be injected i.v. and i.m. (but not s.c.), 250 mg oral/i.m./i.v.; DERIPHYLLIN 100 mg tab., 300 mg SR tab., 220 mg/2 ml inj.

9. **Choline theophyllinate (Oxtriphylline; 64% theophylline):** 250–500 mg oral;
CHOLIPHYLLINE 125 mg cap., 125 mg/5 ml elixir.
10. **Theophylline ethanolate of piperazine:** 250–500 mg oral or i.v.;
CADIPHYLLATE, 80 mg/5 ml elixir; ETOPHYLATE 125 mg/5 ml syrup.
11. **Doxophylline:** 400 mg OD-BD, Children 12 mg/kg/day; DOXORIL 400 mg tab, 100 mg/5 ml syr.
12. **Ipratropium bromide:** 40–80 μg by inhalation; IPRAVENT 20 μg/puff metered dose inhaler, 2 puffs 3–4 times daily; 250 μg/ml respirator soln., 0.4–2 ml nebulized in conjunction with a β_2 agonist 2–4 times daily.
13. **Tiotropium bromide:** 18 μg by inhalation; TIOVA 18 μg rotacaps; 1 rotacap by inhalation OD.
14. **Montelukast:** 10 mg OD; children 2–5 yr 4 mg OD, 6–14 yr 5 mg OD in the evening;
EMLUKAST, MONTAIR, VENTAIR 4 mg, 5 mg, 10 mg tabs.
15. **Zafirlukast:** 20 mg BD; children 5–11 yr 10 mg BD;
ZUVAIR 10 mg, 20 mg tabs.
16. **Sodium cromoglycate:** 2–10 mg by inhalation 3–4 times a day;
FINTAL inhaler: 1 mg metered dose aerosol; 2 puffs 4 times daily.
CROMAL-5 INHALER: 5 mg metered dose aerosol, 2 puffs 4 times daily.
17. **Ketotifen:** 1–2 mg BD; children 0.5 mg BD; ASTHAFEN 1 mg tab, 1 mg/5 ml syrup; KETOVENT 1 mg tab.
18. **Beclomethasone dipropionate:** Initially 100–200 μg BD by inhalation, increase as needed upto 400 μg QID;
BECLATE INHALER 50 μg, 100 μg, 200 μg per metered dose, 200 doses inhaler, BECORIDE 50, 100, 250 μg per puff inhaler.
BECLATE ROTACAPS (with rotahaler) 100, 200, 400 μg powder per cap.
AEROCORT INHALER 50 μg/metered aerosol dose with salbutamol 100 μg.
AEROCORT ROTACAPS 100 μg with salbutamol 200 μg rotacaps (with rotahaler).
19. **Budesonide:** 200–400 μg BD–QID by inhalation in asthma; 200–400 μg/day by intranasal spray for allergic rhinitis.

PULMICORT 100, 200, 400 μg/metered dose inhaler, BUDECORT 100 μg/metered dose inhaler.
FORACORT: Formoterol 6 μg + Budesonide 100 μg/200 μg rotacaps.
RHINOCORT 50 μg per metered dose nasal spray; BUDENASE AQ 100 μg/metered dose aqueous nasal spray; for prophylaxis and treatment of seasonal and perennial allergic or vasomotor rhinitis, nasal polyposis; initially 2 puffs in each nostril every morning, maintenance 1 puff in each nostril in the morning.

20. **Fluticasone propionate:** 100–250 μg BD (max 1000 μg/day) by inhalation; FLOHALE INHALER 25 μg, 50 μg, 125 μg per actuation, FLOHALE ROTACAPS 50 μg, 100 μg, 250 μg rotacaps.
FLOMIST 50 μg per actuation nasal spray.
21. **Flunisolide:** 25 μg by local spray in each nostril BD-TDS;
SYNTARIS 25 μg per actuation nasal spray (for allergic rhinitis).
22. **Ciclesonide:** 80–160 μg by inhalation OD in the evening; CICLEZ 80 μg and 160 μg per metered dose inhaler.

Note: For preparations of systemic corticosteroids, *see* Index.

Some combined antiasthma formulations

BRONKOPLUS: Salbutamol 2 mg, anhydrous theophylline 100 mg tab., also per 5 ml syrup.
BRONKOTUS: Bromhexine 8 mg, salbutamol 2 mg tab., also syrup—bromhexine 4 mg, salbutamol 2 mg per 5 ml.
DUOLIN INHALER, COMBIMIST INHALER Salbutamol 100 μg + ipratropium 20 μg per metered dose inhaler.
DUOLIN ROTACAP salbutamol 200 μg + ipratropium 40 μg per rotacap.
DUOLIN RESPULES, COMBIMIST RESPULES salbutamol 2.5 mg + ipratropium 500 μg in 2.5 ml respirator solution.
TERPHYLIN: Terbutaline 2.5 mg, etophylline 100 mg tab.
THEO ASTHALIN: Salbutamol 2 mg, theophylline anhydrous 100 mg tab.
THEO ASTHALIN-SR: Salbutamol 4 mg, theophylline 300 mg SR tab, also syrup—Salbutamol 2 mg, theophylline 100 mg per 10 ml.
THEOBRIC: Terbutaline 2.5 mg, theophylline 100 mg tab.
THEOBRIC SR: Terbutaline 5 mg, theophylline 300 mg SR tab.

4 Hormones and Related Drugs

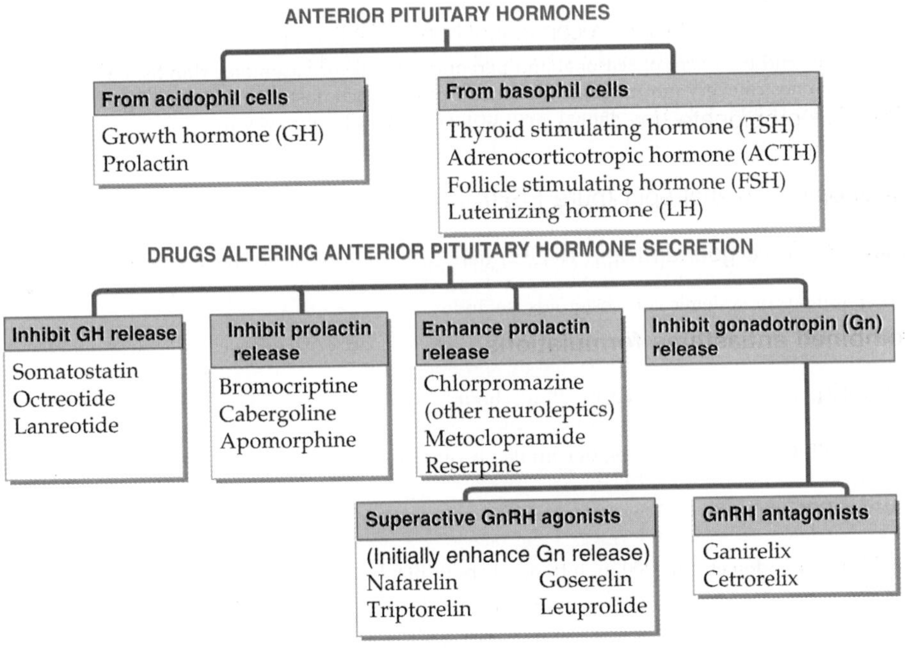

Preparations

1. **Growth hormone (Somatropin: recombinant human GH):** For pituitary dwarfism: 0.03–0.06 mg/kg s.c./i.m. in the evening daily or on alternate days. For adult GH deficiency 150–300 μg/day s.c., later adjusted according to response; NORDITROPIN 5,10,15 mg inj., HUMATROPE 6 mg, 12 mg cartridges, 1.33 and 5.33 mg vials.
2. **Menotropins (FSH + LH):** obtained from urine of menopausal women: PREGNORM, PERGONAL, GYNOGEN 75/150; 75 IU FSH + 75 IU LH activity per amp, also 150 IU FSH + 150 IU LH per amp.
3. **Urofollitropin or Menotropin (pure FSH):** METRODIN, FOLIGEST, FOLICULIN, PUREGON 75 IU and 150 IU per amp.
4. **Human chorionic gonadotropin (HCG)** derived from urine of pregnant women. CORION, PROFASI, PUBERGEN 1000 IU, 2000 IU, 5000 IU, 10,000 IU, all as dry powder with separate solvent for injection.
5. **Somatostatin:** For upper g.i.bleeding 250 μg slow i.v. injection over 3 min followed by 3 mg i.v. infusion over 12 hours. STILMEN, SOMATOSAN, SOMASTAT 250 μg and 3 mg amps.
6. **Octreotide:** 100 μg i.v. followed by 25 μg/hour; SANDOSTATIN, OCTRIDE 50 μg, 100 μg in 1 ml amp, SANDOSTATIN LAR (microsphere formulation) 20 mg/5 ml inj.
7. **Bromocriptine:** Start with 1.25 mg BD, titrate upward upto 10 mg BD; PROCTINAL, PARLODEL, SICRIPTIN, BROMOGEN 1.25 mg, 2.5 mg tabs.
8. **Cabergoline:** Start with 0.25 mg twice weekly, increase upto 1 mg twice weekly as needed; CABERLIN 0.5 mg tab, CAMFORTE 0.5, 1 mg tabs.
9. **Nafarelin:** For endometriosis 200 μg intranasal spray BD; For precocious puberty 800 μg intranasal spray BD; NASAREL 2 mg/ml solution for nasal spray, 200 μg per actuation.

10. **Triptorelin:** For endometriosis and carcinoma prostate: 3.75–7.5 mg of depot injection i.m. every 4 weeks;
For female infertility: 0.1 mg s.c. daily for 10 days starting on 2nd day of menstruation;
For precocious puberty: 50 μg/kg i.m. of depot injection every 4 weeks.
DECAPEPTYL DAILY 0.1 mg inj, DECAPEPTYL DEPOT 3.75 mg inj.

11. **Leuprolide:** For palliative treatment of advanced carcinoma prostate—1 mg s.c. OD or 3.75 mg i.m./s.c. once a month of depot preparation; LUPRIDE 1 mg inj, 3.75 mg depot inj, PROGTASE 1 mg/ml inj.

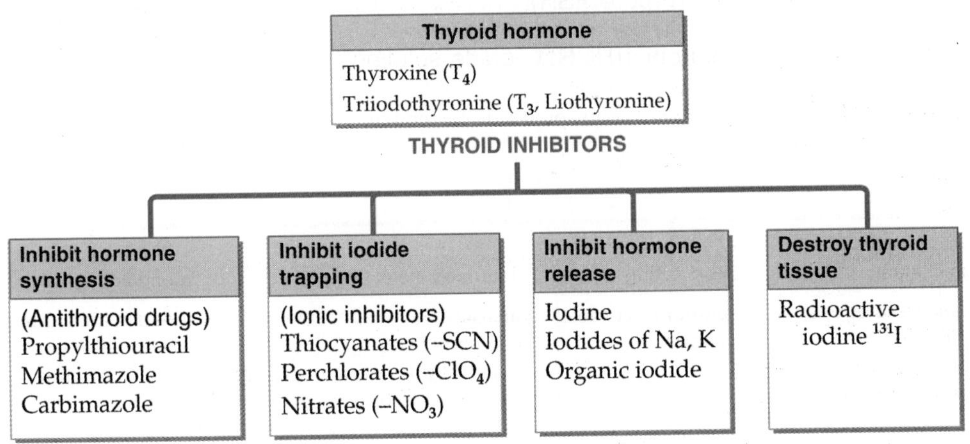

Preparations

L-Thyroxine sod: Adult hypothyroidism—start with 50 μg/day, increase every 2–3 weeks by 25–50 μg to the optimum dose of 100–200 μg/day adjusted by the clinical response and serum TSH level. Cretinism—6–8 μg/kg/day; ELTROXIN, 25, 50, 100 μg tabs, ROXIN 100 μg tab, THYRONORM, 12.5, 25, 50, 62.5, 75, 88, 100, 112, 125, 137, 150 μg tabs, THYROX 25, 50, 75, 100 μg tabs.

1. **Propylthiouracil:** 50–150 mg TDS followed by 25–50 mg BD–TDS for maintenance. PTU 50 mg tab.
2. **Methimazole:** 5–10 mg TDS initially, maintenance dose 5–15 mg daily in 1–2 divided doses.
3. **Carbimazole:** 5–15 mg TDS initially, maintenance dose 2.5–10 mg daily in 1–2 divided doses; NEO MERCAZOLE, THYROZOLE, ANTITHYROX 5 mg tab.
4. **Lugol's solution (5% iodine in 10% Pot. iodide solution):** LUGOL'S SOLUTION, COLLOID IODINE 10%: 5–10 drops/day. COLLOSOL 8 mg iodine/5 ml liq.
5. **Iodide (Sod./Pot.):** 5–10 mg/day prophylactic for endemic goiter; 100–300 mg/day before partial thyroidectomy in Graves' disease.

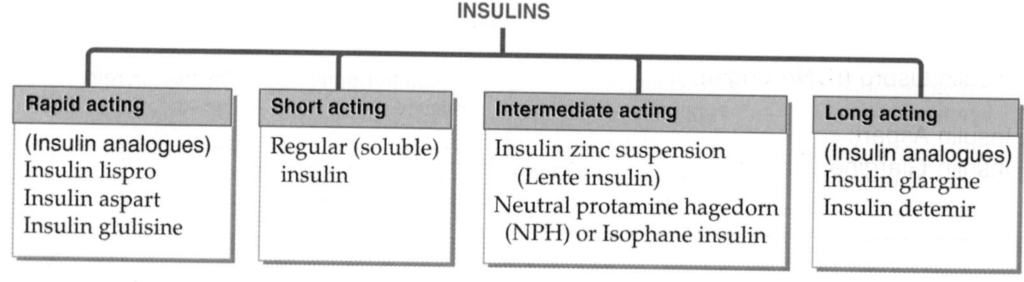

Preparations

(Dose to be individualized according to requirement)

1. ACTRAPID, RAPIDICA: Highly purified pork regular insulin; 40 U/ml.
2. LENTARD, ZINULIN: Highly purified pork lente insulin; 40 U/ml.
3. ACTRAPHANE, RAPIMIX, MIXTARD: Highly purified pork regular insulin (30%) and isophane insulin (70%) 40 U/ml.
4. ACTRAPID MC: Monocomponent pork regular insulin; 40 U/ml, 100 U/ml.
5. MONOTRAD MC: Monocomponent pork lente insulin; 40 U/ml.
6. HUMAN ACTRAPID: Human regular insulin; 40 U/ml, 100 U/ml, ACTRAPID HM PENFIL 100 U/ml pen inj., WOSULIN-R 40 U/ml inj and 100 U/ml pen injector cartridges.
7. HUMAN MONOTRAD, HUMINSULIN-L: Human lente insulin; 40 U/ml, 100 U/ml.
8. HUMAN INSULATARD, HUMINSULIN-N: Human isophane insulin 40 U/ml, WOSULIN-N 40 U/ml inj and 100 U/ml cartridges for pen injector.
9. HUMAN ACTRAPHANE, HUMINSULIN 30/70, HUMAN MIXTARD: Human soluble insulin (30%) and isophane insulin (70%), 40 U/ml, and 100 U/ml vial. WOSULIN-30/70 40 U/ml inj and 100 U/ml cartridges.
10. ACTRAPHANE HM PENFIL: Human soluble insulin 30% + isophane insulin 70% 100 U/ml pen injector.
11. INSUMAN 50/50: Human soluble insulin 50% + isophane insulin 50% 40 U/ml inj; HUMINSULIN 50:50, HUMAN MIXTARD 50; WOSULIN 50/50 40 U/ml inj. and 100 U/ml cartridges.
12. **Insulin Lispro (rDNA origin):** HUMALOG 100 U/ml, 3 ml cartridge and 10 ml vial; to be injected s.c. within 15 min before or immediately after a meal.
13. **Insulin Aspart:** NOVOLOG, NOVORAPID 100 U/ml inj; NOVOMIX 30 FLEXPEN inj (biphasic insulin aspart).
14. **Insulin Glargine:** LANTUS OPTISET 100 U/ml prefilled pen injector 3 ml and vial 5 ml.

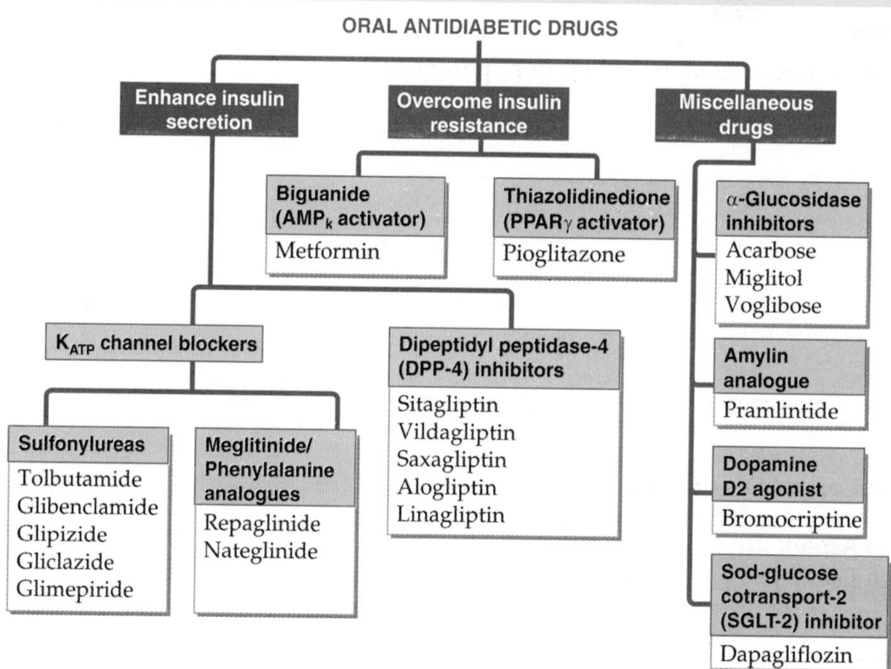
ORAL ANTIDIABETIC DRUGS
Enhance insulin secretion
Overcome insulin resistance
Miscellaneous drugs
Biguanide (AMP_k activator)
Metformin
Thiazolidinedione (PPARγ activator)
Pioglitazone
α-Glucosidase inhibitors
Acarbose
Miglitol
Voglibose
K_{ATP} channel blockers
Dipeptidyl peptidase-4 (DPP-4) inhibitors
Sitagliptin
Vildagliptin
Saxagliptin
Alogliptin
Linagliptin
Amylin analogue
Pramlintide
Sulfonylureas
Tolbutamide
Glibenclamide
Glipizide
Gliclazide
Glimepiride
Meglitinide/ Phenylalanine analogues
Repaglinide
Nateglinide
Dopamine D2 agonist
Bromocriptine
Sod-glucose cotransport-2 (SGLT-2) inhibitor
Dapagliflozin

Preparations

1. **Tolbutamide:** 0.5–3 g/day in 2–3 divided doses; RASTINON 0.5 g tab.
2. **Glibenclamide (Glyburide):** 2.5–15 mg/day in 1–2 doses; DAONIL, EUGLUCON, BETANASE 2.5, 5 mg tab.
3. **Glipizide:** 5–20 mg/day in 1–2 doses; GLYNASE, GLIDE, MINIDIAB 5 mg tab.
4. **Gliclazide:** 40–240 mg/day in 1–2 doses;
   DIAMICRON 80 mg tab, DIAZIDE 20, 80 mg tab, GLIZID 30, 40, 80 mg tab.
5. **Glimepiride:** 1–6 mg per day in 1-2 doses; AMARYL, GLYPRIDE, GLIMER 1, 2 mg tab.
6. **Metformin:** 0.5–2.5 g/day in 1–2 doses; GLYCIPHAGE, GLYCOMET 0.5, 0.85 g tab.
7. **Repaglinide:** 1–8 mg/day in 3–4 doses; EUREPA, REGAN, RAPLIN 0.5, 1, 2 mg tab.
8. **Nateglinide:** 180–480 mg/day in 3–4 doses; GLINATE, NATELIDE 60, 120 mg tab.
9. **Pioglitazone:** 15–45 mg OD; PIONORM, PIOREST, PIOZONE 15, 30 mg tab.
10. **Acarbose:** 50–100 mg TDS taken just before each major meal;
    GLUCOBAY 50, 100 mg tabs, ASUCROSE, GLUCAR 50 mg tab.
11. **Miglitol:** 25-100 mg TDS at beginning of each meal; MIGTOR, DIAMIG, ELITOX 25, 50 mg tab.
12. **Voglibose:** 0.2-0.3 mg TDS just before meals; VOGLITOR, VOLIX, VOLIBO 0.2 and 0.3 mg tabs.
13. **Sitagliptin:** 100 mg OD-BD before meals; JANUVIA 100 mg tab.
14. **Vildagliptin:** 50–100 OD or BD before meals; GALVUS, JALRA, ZOMELIS 50 mg tab.
15. **Saxagliptin:** 5 mg OD; half dose in renal failure; ONGLYZA 2.5, 5 mg tabs.

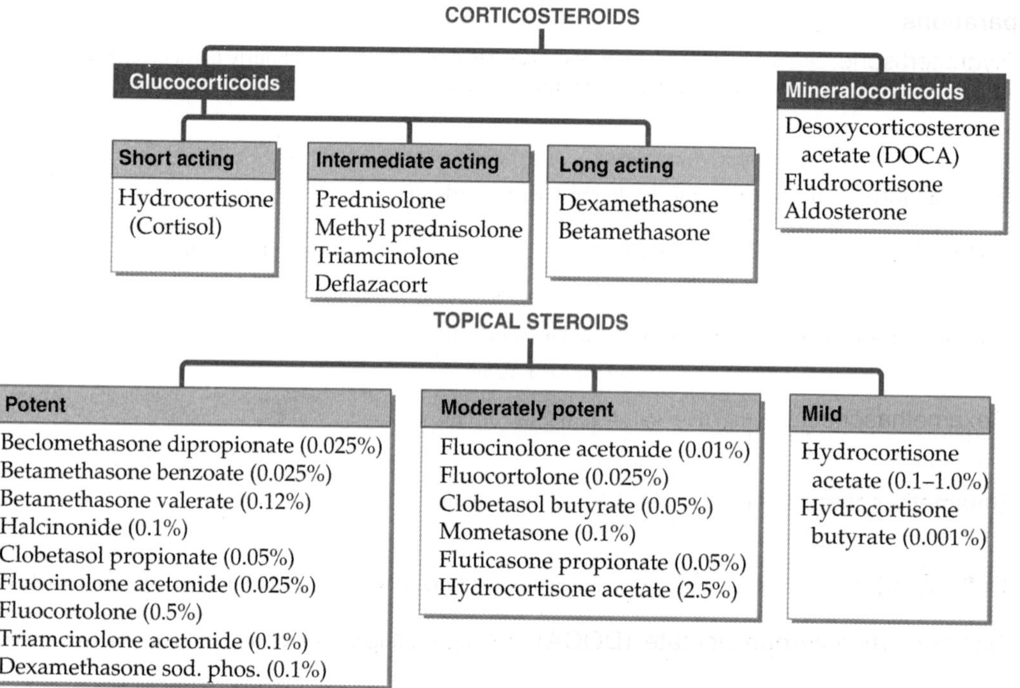
CORTICOSTEROIDS
Glucocorticoids
Short acting
Hydrocortisone (Cortisol)
Intermediate acting
Prednisolone
Methyl prednisolone
Triamcinolone
Deflazacort
Long acting
Dexamethasone
Betamethasone
Mineralocorticoids
Desoxycorticosterone acetate (DOCA)
Fludrocortisone
Aldosterone
TOPICAL STEROIDS
Potent
Beclomethasone dipropionate (0.025%)
Betamethasone benzoate (0.025%)
Betamethasone valerate (0.12%)
Halcinonide (0.1%)
Clobetasol propionate (0.05%)
Fluocinolone acetonide (0.025%)
Fluocortolone (0.5%)
Triamcinolone acetonide (0.1%)
Dexamethasone sod. phos. (0.1%)
Moderately potent
Fluocinolone acetonide (0.01%)
Fluocortolone (0.025%)
Clobetasol butyrate (0.05%)
Mometasone (0.1%)
Fluticasone propionate (0.05%)
Hydrocortisone acetate (2.5%)
Mild
Hydrocortisone acetate (0.1–1.0%)
Hydrocortisone butyrate (0.001%)

Preparations

1. **Hydrocortisone:** 20–30 mg/day oral for replacement therapy; 100 mg i.v. 8 hourly (as hemisuccinate); 100–200 mg i.m./intraarticular (as acetate), 2.0 g as retention enema;
   LYCORTIN-S, EFCORLIN SOLUBLE 100 mg/2 ml vial (as hemisuccinate for i.v. inj.) WYCORT, EFCORLIN 25 mg/ml vial (as acetate for i.m./intraarticualr inj.). PRIMACORT 100, 200, 400 mg/vial inj; ENTOFOAM 2 g in 20 g foam cream (10%) for retention enema.
2. **Prednisolone:** 5–60 mg/day oral, 10–40 mg i.m./intraarticular; DELTACORTRIL, HOSTACORTIN-H, 5, 10 mg tab, 20 mg/ml (as acetate) for i.m., intraarticular inj., WYSOLONE, NUCORT, 5, 10, 20, 40 mg tab.
3. **Methyl prednisolone:** 4–32 mg/day oral, 0.5–1.0 g slow i.v. injection for pulse therapy;
   SOLU-MEDROL methylprednisolone (as sod. succinate) 4 mg tab; 40 mg, 125 mg, 0.5 g (8 ml) and 1.0 g (16 ml) vial, for i.m. or slow i.v. inj., DEESOLONE 4 mg, 16 mg tab, 0.5 g, 1.0 g inj.
4. **Triamcinolone:** 4–32 mg/day oral, 5–40 mg i.m./intraarticular;
   KENACORT, TRICORT 1, 4, 8 mg tab., 10 mg/ml, 40 mg/ml (as acetonide) for i.m., intraarticular inj., LEDERCORT 4 mg tab., KENALOG-S EYE 0.1% with neomycin 0.25% and gramicidin 0.025% eye oint.
5. **Dexamethasone:** 0.5–5 mg/day oral, 4–20 mg i.v. or i.m.;
   DECADRON, DEXONA 0.5 mg tab, 4 mg/ml (as sod. phosphate) for i.v., i.m. inj, 0.5 mg/ml oral drops; WYMESONE, DECDAN 0.5 mg tab, 4 mg/ml inj, OCUDEX, MINIDEX, DEXONA 0.1% eye drops.
6. **Betamethasone:** 0.5–5 mg/day oral, 4–20 mg i.v./i.m. inj;
   BETNESOL, BETACORTRIL, CELESTONE 0.5 mg, 1 mg tab, 4 mg/ml (as sod. phosphate) for i.v., i.m. inj., 0.5 mg/ml oral drops. BETNELAN 0.5 mg, 1 mg tabs, BETNESOL EYE/EAR 0.1% drops and oint.
7. **Deflazacort:** Initially 60–120 mg/day, maintenance 6–18 mg/day, children 0.25–1.5 mg/kg on alternate days. DEFLAR, DEFZA, DFZ 1, 6, 30 mg tabs, DEFGLU 6, 30 mg tabs.
8. **Desoxycorticosterone acetate (DOCA):** 2–5 mg sublingual, 10–20 mg i.m. once or twice weekly; in DOCABOLIN 10 mg/ml inj. (along with nandrolone).

9. Fludrocortisone: Replacement therapy in Addison's disease 50–200 μg daily. Congenital adrenal hyperplasia in patients with salt wasting 50–200 μg/day.

   Idiopathic postural hypotension 100–200 μg/day. FLORICORT 100 μg tab.

Topical Steroids

1. Beclomethasone dipropionate 0.025% BECLATE cream
2. Betamethasone benzoate 0.025% TOPICASONE cream, oint.
3. Betamethasone valerate 0.12% BETNOVATE cream, oint., BETASONE cream
4. Halcinonide 0.1% CORTILATE, HALOG cream
5. Clobetasol propionate 0.05% LOBATE, TENOVATE, DERMOTYL cream
6. Dexamethasone sod. phosphate 0.1% DECADRON cream (with Neomycin 0.35%)
7. Dexamethasone trimethyl-acetate 0.1% MILLICORTENOL cream
8. Fluocinolone acetonide 0.025% FLUCORT oint., LUCI oint.
9. Fluocortolone 0.5% ULTRALAN oint.
10. Triamcinolone acetonide 0.1% LEDERCORT oint.
11. Fluocinolone acetonide 0.01% FLUCORT-H oint. and skin lotion
12. Clobetasol butyrate 0.05% EUMOSONE cream
13. Fluocortolone 0.25% COLSIPAN oint.
14. Mometasone 0.1% MOMATE, CUTIZONE oint, cream
15. Fluticasone propionate 0.05% FLUTIVATE, MOLIDERM cream
16. Hydrocortisone + (urea 12%) 1% COTARYL-H cream.
17. Hydrocortisone acetate 2.5% WYCORT oint.

18. **Hydrocortisone acetate** 0.1–1.0% LYCORTIN 1% oint., in CORTOQUINOL 1% with quiniodochlor, 4% cream, GENTACYN-HC TOPICAL 1% with gentamicin 0.1%, CORTISON-KEMICETINE 0.5% with chloramphenicol 0.5%.
19. **Hydrocortisone butyrate** 0.001% LOCOID cream

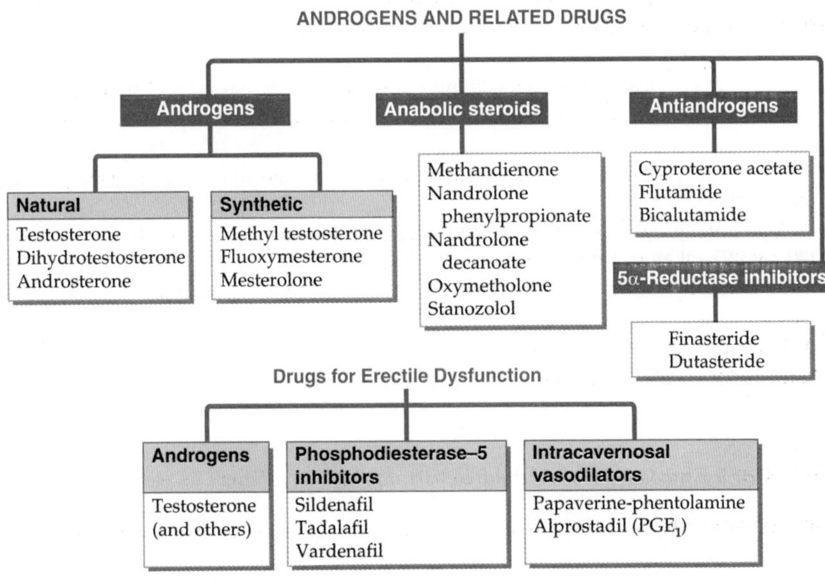

Preparations

Androgens

1. **Testosterone (free):** 25 mg i.m. daily to twice weekly; AQUAVIRON 25 mg in 1 ml inj.
2. **Testosterone propionate:** 25–50 mg i.m. daily to twice weekly; TESTOVIRON, PARENDREN, TESTANON 25, 50 mg/ml inj.
3. TESTOVIRON DEPOT 100: testo. propionate 25 mg + testo. enanthate 100 mg in 1 ml amp; 1 ml i.m. weekly.
4. TESTOVIRON DEPOT 250: testo. propionate 250 mg + testo. enanthate 250 mg in 1 ml amp; 1 ml i.m. every 2–4 weeks.
5. SUSTANON '100': testo. propionate 20 mg + testo. phenyl propionate 40 mg + testo. isocaproate 40 mg in 1 ml amp; 1 ml i.m. every 2–3 weeks.
6. SUSTANON '250': testo. propionate 30 mg + testo. phenylpropionate 60 mg + testo. isocaproate 60 mg + testo. decanoate 100 mg in 1 ml amp; 1 ml i.m. every 3–4 weeks.
7. **Testosterone undecanoate:** NUVIR, ANDRIOL; 40 mg cap, 1–3 cap daily for male hypogonadism, osteoporosis.
8. **Mesterolone:** 25 mg OD–TDS oral; PROVIRONUM, RESTORE, MESTILON 25 mg tab.
9. **Dihydrotestosterone:** 100–250 mg cutaneous application daily; ANDRACTIM 25 mg/g gel for application over nonscrotal skin once daily.

Anabolic Steroids

10. **Methandienone:** 2–5 mg OD–BD oral; children 0.04 mg/kg/day, 25 mg i.m. weekly; ANABOLEX 2, 5 mg tab, 2 mg/ml drops, 25 mg/ml inj.
11. **Nandrolone phenyl propionate:** 10–50 mg; children 10 mg; i.m. once or twice weekly; DURABOLIN 10, 25 mg/ml inj.

12. **Nandrolone decanoate:** 25–100 mg i.m. every 3 weeks, DECADURABOLIN 25, 100 mg/ml inj.
13. **Oxymetholone:** 5–10 mg, children 0.1 mg/kg, OD; ADROYD 5 mg tab.
14. **Stanozolol:** 2–6 mg/day; MENABOL, NEURABOL, TANZOL 2 mg tab.

Impeded Androgen

15. **Danazol:** 200–600 mg/day; DANAZOL, LADOGAL, DANOGEN, GONABLOK 50, 100, 200 mg cap.

Antiandrogens

16. **Cyproterone acetate:** 2 mg OD; GINETTE-35, DINAC-35 (cyproterone acetate 2 mg + ethinylestradiol 35 μg) tab.
17. **Flutamide:** 250 mg TDS; PROSTAMID, FLUTIDE, CYTOMID 250 mg tab.
18. **Bicalutamide:** 50 mg OD; BIPROSTA, CALUTIDE, TABI 50 mg tab.

5α-Reductase Inhibitor

19. **Finasteride:** For benign hypertrophy of prostate (BHP) 5 mg OD, review after 6 months; for male pattern baldness 1 mg/day. FINCAR, FINARA, FINAST 5 mg tab, FINPECIA, ASTIFINE 1 mg tab.
20. **Dutasteride:** For BHP 0.5 mg/day. DUPROST, DURIZE 0.5 mg tab.

Drugs for Erectile Dysfunction

1. **Sildenafil:** 50 mg (max. 100 mg) 1 hour before intercourse; elderly 25 mg;
   PENEGRA, CAVERTA, EDEGRA 25, 50, 100 mg tabs.
2. **Tadalafil:** 10 mg (max. 20 mg) at least ½ hr before intercourse.
   MEGALIS, TADARICH, TADALIS 10, 20 mg tab, MANFORCE 10 mg tab.

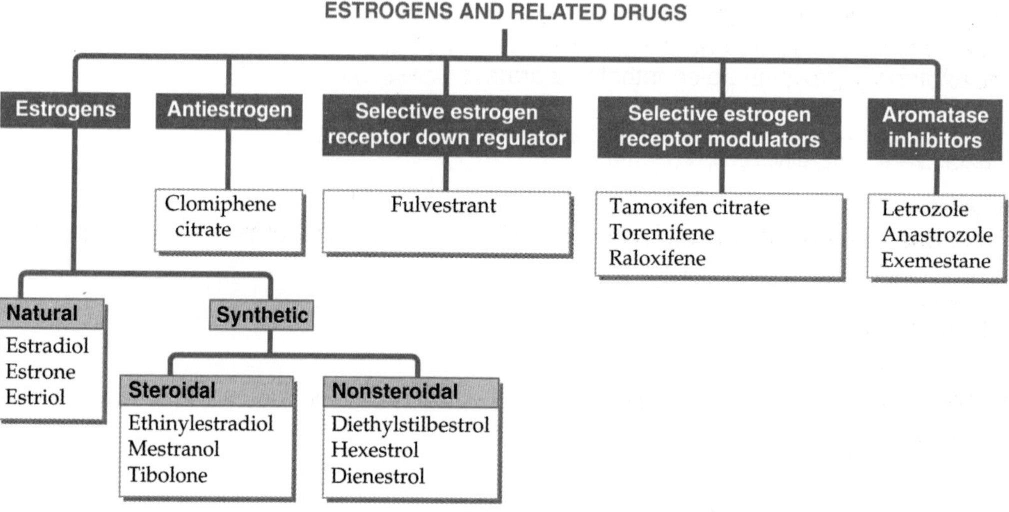
ESTROGENS AND RELATED DRUGS
Estrogens
Antiestrogen
Selective estrogen receptor down regulator
Selective estrogen receptor modulators
Aromatase inhibitors
Clomiphene citrate
Fulvestrant
Tamoxifen citrate
Toremifene
Raloxifene
Letrozole
Anastrozole
Exemestane
Natural
Estradiol
Estrone
Estriol
Synthetic
Steroidal
Ethinylestradiol
Mestranol
Tibolone
Nonsteroidal
Diethylstilbestrol
Hexestrol
Dienestrol

Preparations

Estrogens

1. Estradiol benzoate/cypionate/enanthate/valarate: 2.5–10 mg i.m.; OVOCYCLIN-P 5 mg inj, PROGYNON DEPOT 10 mg/ml inj.
2. Conjugated estrogens: 0.625–1.25 mg/day oral for hormone replacement therapy; PREMARIN 0.625 mg, 1.25 mg tab, 25 mg inj (for dysfunctional uterine bleeding).
3. Ethinylestradiol: for menopausal syndrome 0.02–0.2 mg/day oral; LYNORAL 0.01, 0.05, 1.0 mg tab, PROGYNON-C 0.02 mg tab.
4. Mestranol: 0.1–0.2 mg/day oral; in OVULEN 0.1 mg tab, with ethynodiol diacetate 1 mg.
5. Estriol succinate: 4–8 mg/day initially, maintenance dose in menopause 1–2 mg/day oral; EVALON 1, 2 mg tab, 1 mg/g cream for vaginal application in atrophic vaginitis 1–3 times daily.
6. Fosfestrol tetrasodium: initially 600–1200 mg slow i.v. inj for 5 days, maintenance dose 120–240 mg/day oral or 300 mg 1–3 times a week i.v.; HONVAN 120 mg tab, 60 mg/ml inj 5 ml amp.
7. Dienestrol: 0.01% topical; DIENESTROL 0.01% vaginal cream.
8. Estradiol transdermal: ESTRADERM-MX: Estradiol 25, 50 or 100 μg per 24 hr transdermal patches; apply to nonhairy skin below waist, replace every 3–4 days using a different site; add an oral progestin for last 10–12 days every month.
9. Estradiol dermal gel: 1–2.5 mg/day; OESTRAGEL, E_2GEL 3 mg/5 g gel in 80 g tube, SANDRENA 1 mg/g gel; apply 1.5–4 g gel over arms & shoulder daily.
10. Tibolone: 2.5 mg/day without interruption in postmenopausal women; LIVIAL, TIBOFEM 2.5 mg tab.

Antiestrogen

Clomiphene citrate: for infertility in women—50 mg/day for 5 days starting from 5th day of cycle, increase to 100 mg/day after 2–3 unsuccessful cycles (max. 200 mg/day); for oligozoospermia in men—25 mg daily for 24 days in a month upto 6 months; CLOMID, FERTOMID, CLOFERT, CLOME 25, 50, 100 mg tabs.

Selective Estrogen Receptor Down Regulator/Pure Estrogen Antagonist

Fulvestrant: 250 mg i.m. (in gluteal region) monthly.

Selective Estrogen Receptor Modulators (SERMs)

1. Tamoxifen citrate: 20 mg/day in 1–2 doses (max. 40 mg/day).
   TAMOXIFEN, MAMOFEN, TAMODEX 10, 20 mg tabs.
2. Toremifene: 60 mg OD.
3. Raloxifene: 60 mg/day; OSRAL, BONMAX, RALOTAB, ESSERM 60 mg tab.

Aromatase Inhibitors

1. Letrozole: 2.5 mg/day oral; FEMARA, ONCOLET, LETOVAL, LETROZ 2.5 mg tab.
2. Anastrozole: 1 mg/day oral; ARMOTRAZ, ALTRAZ, ANABREZ 1 mg tab.
3. Exemestane: 25 mg/day oral.

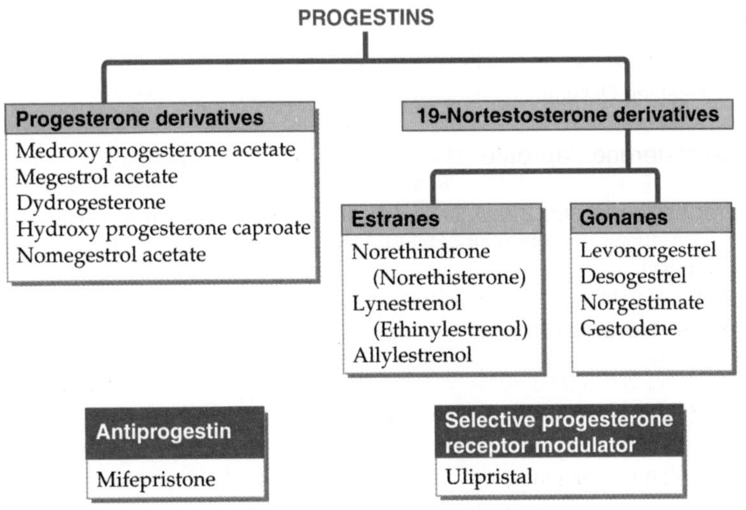
PROGESTINS
Progesterone derivatives
Medroxy progesterone acetate
Megestrol acetate
Dydrogesterone
Hydroxy progesterone caproate
Nomegestrol acetate
19-Nortestosterone derivatives
Estranes
Norethindrone
(Norethisterone)
Lynestrenol
(Ethinylestrenol)
Allylestrenol
Gonanes
Levonorgestrel
Desogestrel
Norgestimate
Gestodene
Antiprogestin
Mifepristone
Selective progesterone receptor modulator
Ulipristal

Preparations

1. **Progesterone:** 10–100 mg i.m. (as oily solution) OD; PROGEST, PROLUTON, GESTONE 50 mg/ml inj., 1 and 2 ml amp; 100–400 mg OD oral: NATUROGEST, OGEST, DUBAGEST 100, 200, 400 mg caps containing micronized oily suspension.
2. **Hydroxyprogesterone caproate:** 250–500 mg i.m. at 2–14 days intervals; PROLUTON DEPOT, MAINTANE INJ, PROCAPRIN 250 mg/ml in 1 and 2 ml amp.
3. **Medroxyprogesterone acetate:** 5–20 mg OD–BD oral, 50–150 mg i.m. at 1–3 month interval; FARLUTAL 2.5, 5, 10 mg tab., PROVERA, MEPRATE, MODUS 10 mg tab, DEPOT-PROVERA 150 mg in 1 ml inj. (as contraceptive).
4. **Dydrogesterone:** 5–10 mg OD/TDS oral; DUPHASTON 5 mg tab.
5. **Norethindrone (Norethisterone):** 5–10 mg OD–BD oral; PRIMOLUT-N, STYPTIN, REGESTRONE, NORGEST 5 mg tab; REGESTRONE HRT, NORETA HRT 1 mg tab (for HRT); NORISTERAT 200 mg/ml inj (as enanthate) for contraception 1 ml i.m every 2 months.
6. **Lynestrenol (Ethinylestrenol):** 5–10 mg OD oral; ORGAMETRIL 5 mg tab.
7. **Allylestrenol:** 10–40 mg/day; GESTANIN, FETUGARD, MAINTANE 5 mg tab, PROFAR 25 mg tab.
8. **Levonorgestrel:** 0.1–0.5 mg/day; DUOLUTON-L, OVRAL 0.25 mg + ethinylestradiol 0.05 mg tab.
9. **Desogestrel:** 150 μg + ethinylestradiol 30 μg (NOVELON) tab, 1 tab OD, 3 weeks on and 1 week off cyclic therapy.

Antiprogestin

Mifepristone: 200–600 mg single oral dose; MIFEGEST, MIFEPRIN 200 mg tab.

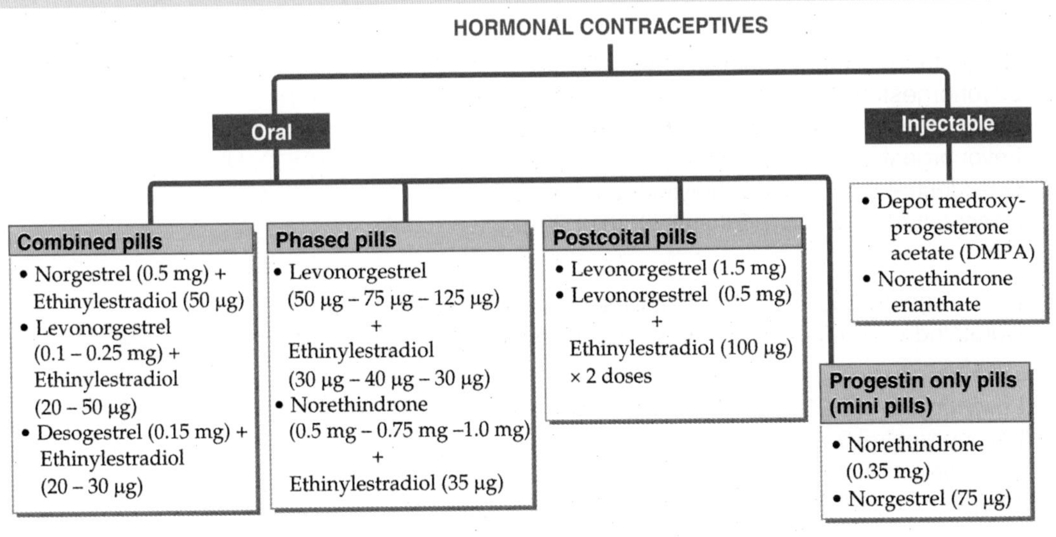
HORMONAL CONTRACEPTIVES
Oral
Injectable
Combined pills
• Norgestrel (0.5 mg) + Ethinylestradiol (50 μg)
• Levonorgestrel (0.1 – 0.25 mg) + Ethinylestradiol (20 – 50 μg)
• Desogestrel (0.15 mg) + Ethinylestradiol (20 – 30 μg)
Phased pills
• Levonorgestrel (50 μg – 75 μg – 125 μg) + Ethinylestradiol (30 μg – 40 μg – 30 μg)
• Norethindrone (0.5 mg – 0.75 mg –1.0 mg) + Ethinylestradiol (35 μg)
Postcoital pills
• Levonorgestrel (1.5 mg)
• Levonorgestrel (0.5 mg) + Ethinylestradiol (100 μg) × 2 doses
Progestin only pills (mini pills)
• Norethindrone (0.35 mg)
• Norgestrel (75 μg)
• Depot medroxy-progesterone acetate (DMPA)
• Norethindrone enanthate

Combined Pills

1. Norgestrel 0.5 mg + Ethinylestradiol 50 μg; OVRAL-G, 20 tabs.
2. Levonorgestrel 0.25 mg + Ethinylestradiol 50 μg; OVRAL, DUOLUTON-L, 21 tabs.
3. Levonorgestrel 0.15 mg + Ethinylestradiol 30 μg; OVRAL-L, OVIPAUZ, 21 tabs.
4. Levonorgestrel 0.1 mg + Ethinylestradiol 20 μg; LOETTE, OVILOW, COMBEE 21 tabs.
5. Desogestrel 0.15 mg + Ethinylestradiol 30 μg; NOVELON.
6. Desogestrel 0.15 mg + Ethinylestradiol 20 μg; FEMILON.

Phased Pills

1. Levonorgestrel 50–75–125 μg + Ethinylestradiol 30–40–30 μg; TRIQUILAR (6 + 5 + 10 tablets)
2. Norethindrone 0.5–0.75–1.0 mg + Ethinylestradiol 35–35–35 μg; ORTHONOVUM 7/7/7 tabs.

Postcoital Pills

1. Levonorgestrel 0.25 mg + Ethinylestradiol 50 μg; OVRAL, DUOLUTON-L (2 + 2 tabs)
2. Levonorgestrel 0.75 mg; NORLEVO, ECEE2 (1 + 1 tab)
3. Levonorgestrel 1.5 mg iPILL, NOFEAR-72 (1 tab).
4. Mifepristone 600 mg; MIFEGEST, MIFEPRIN 200 mg (3 tabs)
5. Ulipristal (selective progesterone receptor modulator) 30 mg single dose as soon as possible, before 120 hours of intercourse.

Mini Pills

1. Norethindrone 0.35 mg
2. Norgestrel 75 μg

Anti implantation SERM

Centchroman (Ormeloxifene): 30 mg twice weekly for 12 weeks and then 30 mg weekly; CENTRON, SAHELI 30 mg tab.

Injectable Contraceptives

1. **Depot medroxyprogesterone acetate (DMPA):** 150 mg i.m. at 3 month intervals.
   DEPOT-PROVERA 150 mg in 1 ml vial for deep i.m. injection during first 5 days of menstrual cycle. Repeat every 3 months.
2. **Norethindrone (Norethisterone) enanthate (NEE):** 200 mg i.m. at 2 month intervals.
   NORISTERAT 200 mg in 1 ml vial for deep i.m. injection during first 5 days of menstrual cycle. Repeat every 2 months.

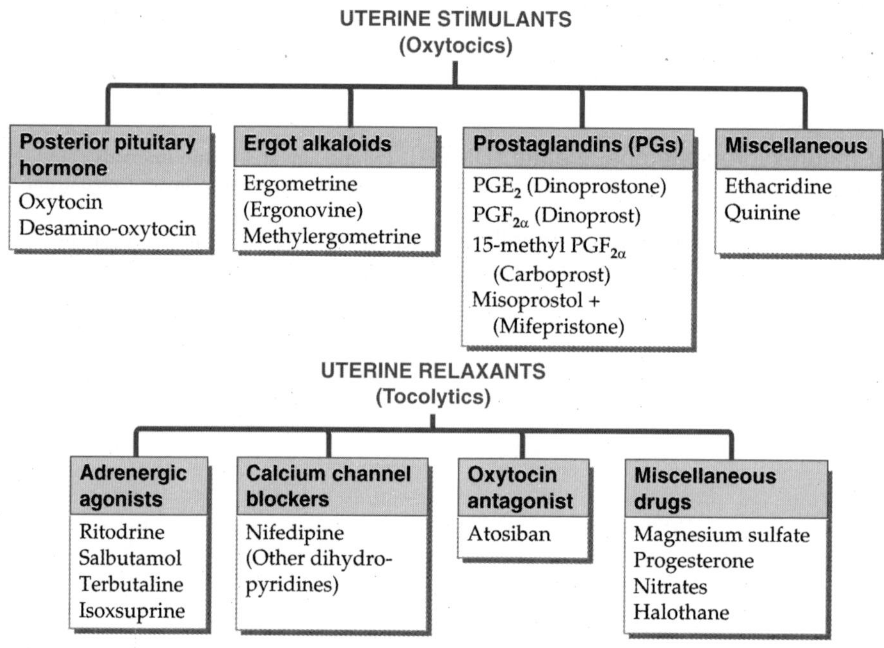

UTERINE STIMULANTS
(Oxytocics)
Posterior pituitary hormone
Oxytocin
Desamino-oxytocin
Ergot alkaloids
Ergometrine (Ergonovine)
Methylergometrine
Prostaglandins (PGs)
PGE_2 (Dinoprostone)
$PGF_{2\alpha}$ (Dinoprost)
15-methyl $PGF_{2\alpha}$ (Carboprost)
Misoprostol + (Mifepristone)
Miscellaneous
Ethacridine
Quinine
UTERINE RELAXANTS
(Tocolytics)
Adrenergic agonists
Ritodrine
Salbutamol
Terbutaline
Isoxsuprine
Calcium channel blockers
Nifedipine
(Other dihydro-pyridines)
Oxytocin antagonist
Atosiban
Miscellaneous drugs
Magnesium sulfate
Progesterone
Nitrates
Halothane

Preparations

Uterine Stimulants

1. **Oxytocin:** for induction/augmentation of labour 2–10 milli IU/min i.v. infusion (total 2–4 IU); for postpartum haemorrhage 5 IU i.m. or i.v. infusion;
   OXYTOCIN, SYNTOCINON 2 IU/2 ml and 5 IU/ml inj., PITOCIN 5 IU/0.5 ml inj.
2. **Desamino-oxytocin:** for induction 50 IU buccal every 30 min, for uterine inertia 25 IU buccal every 30 min; for breast engorgement 25–50 IU just before breast feeding; BUCTOCIN 50 IU buccal tab.
3. **Ergometrine:** 0.2–0.5 mg i.m./i.v., 0.25–0.5 mg TDS oral; ERGOMETRINE 0.25, 0.5 mg tab, 0.5 mg/ml inj.
4. **Methylergometrine:** 0.2–0.5 mg i.m./i.v., 0.125–0.25 mg TDS oral;
   METHERGIN, METHERONE, ERGOMET 0.125 mg tab, 0.2 mg/ml inj.
5. **Ethacridine:** 150 mg extra-amniotic infusion; EMCREDIL, VECREDIL 50 mg/50 ml inj.

Note: For preparations of prostaglandins and uterine relaxants, *see* Index

5 Drugs Acting on Peripheral (somatic) Nervous System

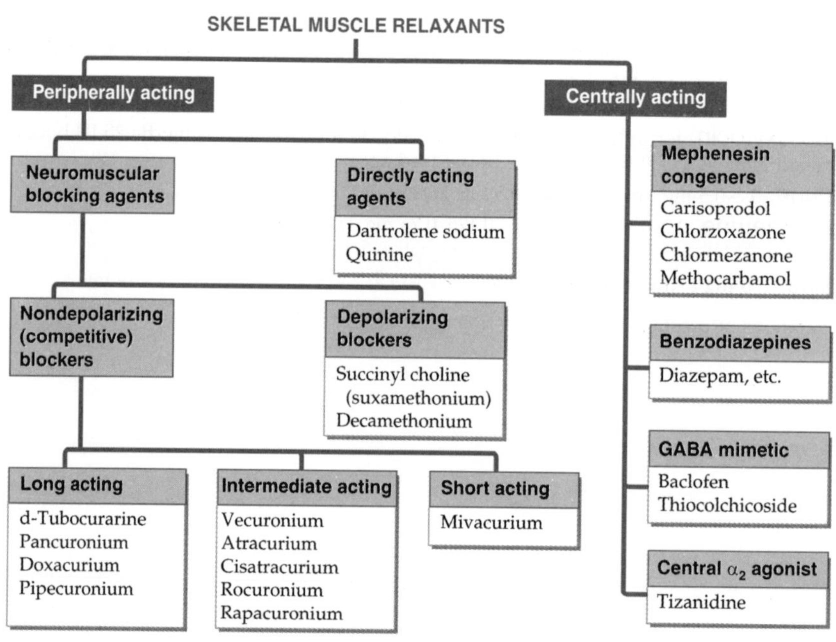

Preparations

(Note: Doses of neuromuscular blocking agents given below are initial paralysing doses for nitrous oxide-oxygen/opioid anaesthesia. These doses are to be reduced to 1/3–1/2 in patients anaesthetised with ether/halothane/isoflurane etc.)

1. **Pancuronium:** 0.04–0.1 mg/kg i.v.; PAVULON, PANURON, NEOCURON 2 mg/ml in 2 ml amp.
2. **Doxacurium:** 0.03–0.08 mg/kg i.v.
3. **Pipecuronium:** 0.05–0.08 mg/kg i.v.; ARDUAN 4 mg/2 ml inj.
4. **Vecuronium:** 0.08–0.1 mg/kg i.v.; NORCURON, NEOVEC 4 mg amp. and 10 mg vial; dissolve in 1–2.5 ml solvent supplied.
5. **Atracurium:** 0.3–0.6 mg/kg i.v.; TACRIUM 10 mg/ml in 2 ml vial.
6. **Cisatracurium:** 0.15–0.2 mg/kg i.v.
7. **Rocuronium:** 0.6–0.9 mg/kg i.v.; CUROMID, ROCUNIUM 50 mg/5 ml, 100 mg/10 ml vials.
8. **Mivacurium:** 0.07–0.15 mg/kg i.v.
9. **Succinylcholine (Suxamethonium):** 0.5–0.8 mg/kg i.v.; MIDARINE, SCOLINE, MYORELEX, ENTUBATE 50 mg/ml in 2 ml amp.
10. **Dantrolene:** 25–100 mg QID oral, 1 mg/kg i.v. repeated as required.
11. **Carisoprodol:** 350 mg TDS–QID oral; CARISOMA 350 mg tab; SOMAFLAM 175 mg + ibuprofen 400 mg tab.
12. **Chlorzoxazone:** 500 mg BD–TDS; ULTRAZOX 250 mg + diclofenac 50 mg + paracetamol 325 mg tab; MOBIZOX 500 mg + diclofenac 50 mg + paracetamol 500 mg tab; PARAFON 250 mg + paracetamol 300 mg tab; FLEXON-MR 250 mg + ibuprofen 400 mg + paracetamol 325 mg tab.
13. **Chlormezanone:** 100–200 mg TDS–QID; DOLOBAK 100 mg + paracetamol 450 mg tab.
14. **Methocarbamol:** 400–800 mg TDS oral, 100–200 mg i.m./i.v.; ROBINAX 0.5 g tab, 1 TDS: 100 mg/ml inj. for i.v. or i.m. use. ROBIFLAM 750 mg + ibuprofen 200 mg tab; NEUROMOL-MR 400 mg + paracetamol 500 mg tab.

15. **Baclofen:** 10 mg BD–25 mg TDS oral; LIORESAL, LIOFEN 10, 25 mg tabs.
16. **Thiocolchicoside:** 4 mg TDS-QID; NUCOXIA-MR: thiocolchicoside 4 mg + etoricoxib 60 mg tabs.
17. **Tizanidine:** 2 mg TDS; max 24 mg/day; SIRDALUD 2, 4, 6 mg tab; TIZAN 2, 4 mg tab; BRUFEN-MR, TIZAFEN 2 mg + ibuprofen 400 mg tab; TIZANAC 2 mg + diclofenac 50 mg tab., PROXYVON-MR 2 mg + nimesulide 100 mg cap.

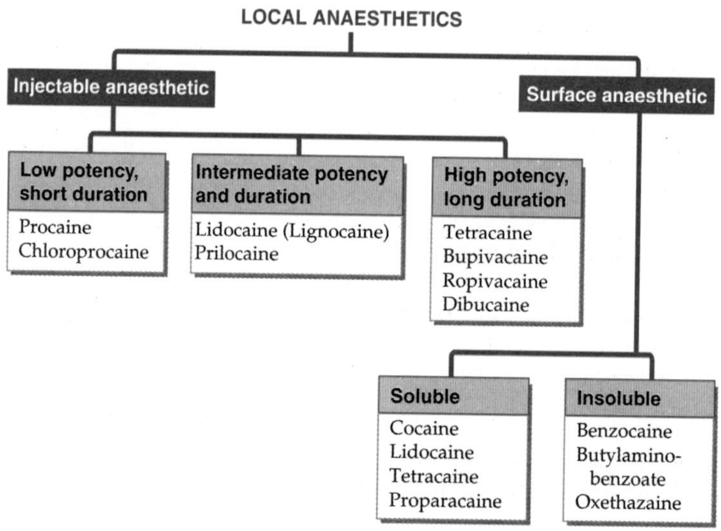

Preparations

1. **Lidocaine (lignocaine):** 0.5–2% for nerve block, 1–5% topically; XYLOCAINE, GESICAIN 4% topical solution, 2% jelly, 2% viscous, 5% ointment, 1% and 2% injection (with or without adrenaline), 5% heavy (for spinal anaesthesia); 100 mg/ml spray (10 mg per puff)
2. **Bupivacaine:** 0.25–0.5% for nerve block, 0.5–0.75% for spinal anaesthesia; MARCAIN 0.5%, 1% (hyperbaric for spinal anaesthesia). SENSORCAINE 0.25%, 0.5% inj, 0.5% heavy inj.
3. **Tetracaine (Amethocaine):** 0.25% for nerve block, 0.25–0.5% for spinal anaesthesia, 1% topically; ANETHANE powder for preparing solution, 1% oint.
4. **Eutectic Lidocaine-prilocaine:** 5% for cutaneous anaesthesia; PRILOX 5% cream
5. **Dibucaine:** 0.25–0.5% for nerve block and spinal anaesthesia, 1% for surface anaesthesia; NUPERCAINE 0.5% inj, NUPERCAINAL 1% oint, in OTOGESIC 1% ear drops.
6. **Benzocaine:** 5–20% topically; in PROCTOQUINOL 5% oint., ZOKEN 20% gel.
7. **Butylaminobenzoate:** 1–5% topically; in PROCTOSEDYL-M 1% oint with framycetin and hydrocortisone for anal application.
8. **Benoxinate:** 0.4% for corneal anaesthesia; BENDZON 0.4% eye drops.
9. **Oxethazaine:** 0.2% for gastric mucosal anaesthesia;
   MUCAINE 0.2% in alumina gel + magnesium hydroxide suspension; 5–10 ml orally.
   TRICAINE-MPS: Oxethazaine 10 mg with methyl polysiloxane 125 mg, alum. hydroxide gel 300 mg, mag. hydroxide 150 mg per 5 ml gel.

6 Drugs Acting on Central Nervous System

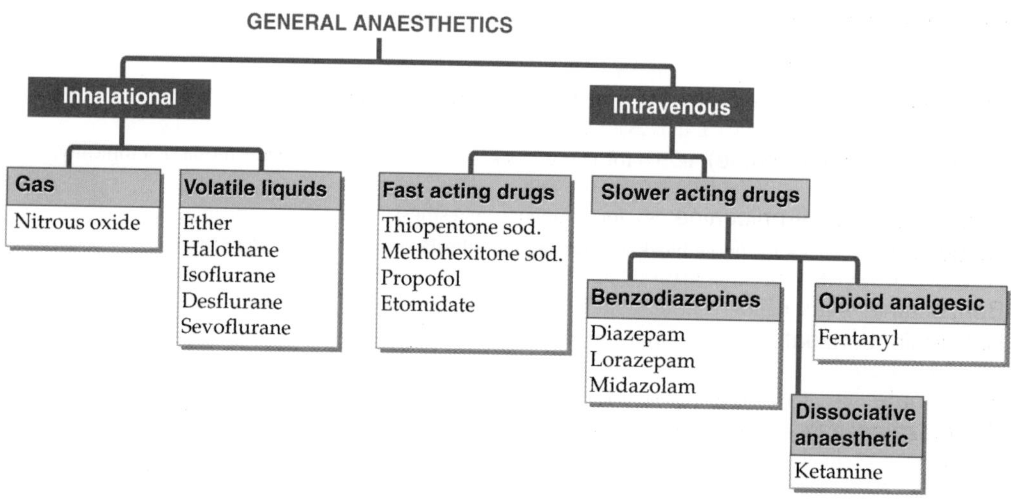

Preparations

1. **Thiopentone sod.:** 3–5 mg/kg i.v. for induction;
   PENTOTHAL, INTRAVAL SODIUM 0.5, 1.0 g for preparing injectable solution freshly.
2. **Propofol:** 2 mg/kg bolus i.v. injection for induction, 9 mg/kg/hr for maintenance;
   PROPOVAN 10 mg/ml and 20 mg/ml in 10, 20 ml vials.
3. **Diazepam:** 0.25–0.5 mg/kg by slow injection in a running i.v. drip; VALIUM, CALMPOSE 10 mg/2 ml inj.
4. **Lorazepam:** 0.04 mg/kg (2–4 mg total for adult) i.v.; CALMESE 4 mg/2 ml inj.
5. **Midazolam:** 1–2.5 mg i.v. bolus injection, 0.02–0.1 mg/kg/hour i.v. infusion for maintenance;
   MEZOLAM, FULSED, SHORTAL 1 mg/ml and 5 mg/ml inj.
6. **Ketamine:** 1–3 mg/kg i.v., 5 mg/kg i.m.; KETMIN, KETAMAX, ANEKET 50 mg/ml in 2 ml amp, 10 ml vial.
7. **Fentanyl:** 2–4 μg/kg i.v.; TROFENTYL, FENT, FENDOP 50 μg/ml in 2 ml amp, 10 ml vial.

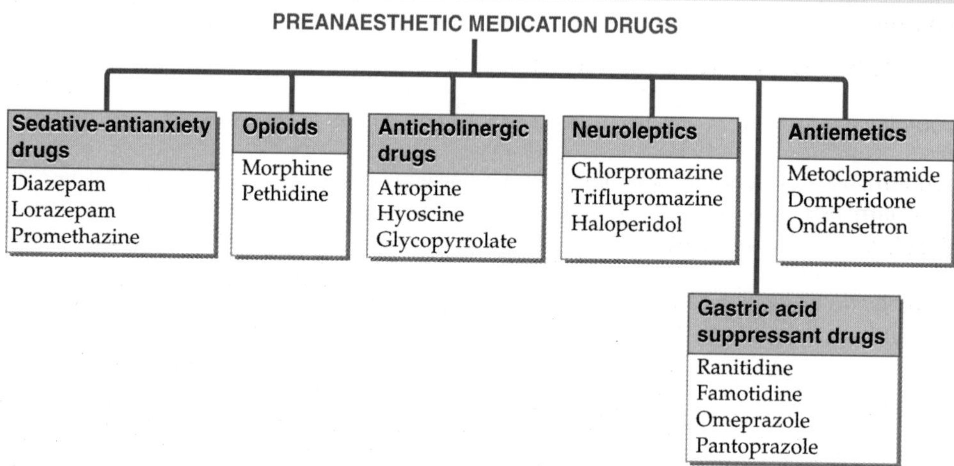

Preanaesthetic Medication Drugs

Note: See Index for preparations

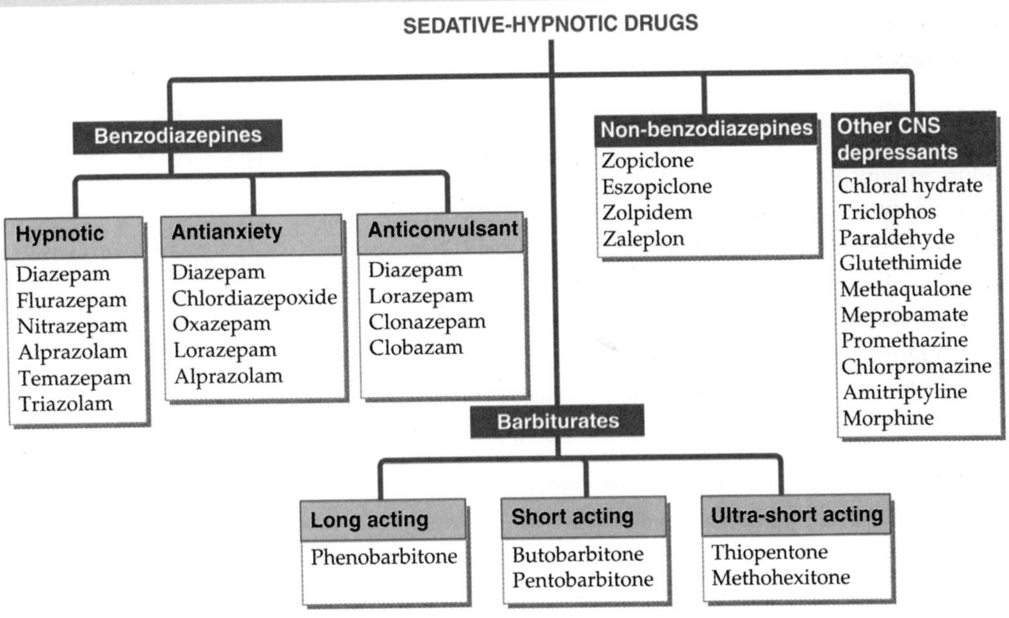
SEDATIVE-HYPNOTIC DRUGS
Benzodiazepines
Hypnotic
Diazepam
Flurazepam
Nitrazepam
Alprazolam
Temazepam
Triazolam
Antianxiety
Diazepam
Chlordiazepoxide
Oxazepam
Lorazepam
Alprazolam
Anticonvulsant
Diazepam
Lorazepam
Clonazepam
Clobazam
Non-benzodiazepines
Zopiclone
Eszopiclone
Zolpidem
Zaleplon
Other CNS depressants
Chloral hydrate
Triclophos
Paraldehyde
Glutethimide
Methaqualone
Meprobamate
Promethazine
Chlorpromazine
Amitriptyline
Morphine
Barbiturates
Long acting
Phenobarbitone
Short acting
Butobarbitone
Pentobarbitone
Ultra-short acting
Thiopentone
Methohexitone

Preparations

1. **Phenobarbitone:** 30–60 mg OD–TDS (as antiepileptic) 100–200 mg i.m./i.v.; GARDENAL 30, 60 mg tab; LUMINAL 30 mg tab; PHENOBARBITONE SOD 200 mg/ml inj.
2. **Diazepam:** 2.5–10 mg (as hypnotic), 5–30 mg/day (as antianxiety); VALIUM 2, 5, 10 mg tab., 10 mg/2 ml inj., CALMPOSE 5, 10 mg tab, 2 mg/5 ml syr, 10 mg/2 ml inj.
3. **Flurazepam:** 15–30 mg (as hypnotic); NINDRAL, FLURAZ 15 mg cap.
4. **Nitrazepam:** 5–10 mg (as hypnotic); SEDAMON, HYPNOTEX, NITRAVET 5, 10 mg tab/cap.
5. **Alprazolam:** 0.25–1.0 mg (hypnotic dose), 0.25–1.0 mg TDS for anxiety; ALPRAX 0.25, 0.5, 1.0 mg tabs., 0.5, 1.0, 1.5 mg SR tabs; ALZOLAM 0.25, 0.5, 1.0 mg tabs; 1.5 mg SR tab, RESTYL 0.25, 0.5, 1.0 mg tab, RESTYL-SR 0.5, 1.0, 1.5 mg SR tab, ALPROCONTIN 0.5, 1.0, 1.5 mg CR tabs.
6. **Temazepam:** 10–20 mg (as hypnotic).
7. **Triazolam:** 0.125–0.25 mg (as hypnotic).
8. **Zopiclone:** 7.5 mg (hypnotic dose), elderly 3.75 mg; ZOPICON, ZOLIUM, ZOPITRAN 7.5 mg tab.
9. **Zolpidem:** 5–10 mg (max 20 mg) as hypnotic; elderly and liver disease patients 2.5–10 mg; NITREST, ZOLDEM, DEM 5, 10 mg tabs.
10. **Zaleplon:** 5–10 mg (max 20 mg) hypnotic dose; ZAPLON, ZASO, ZALEP 5, 10 mg tabs.

Note: See Index for preparations of other drugs.

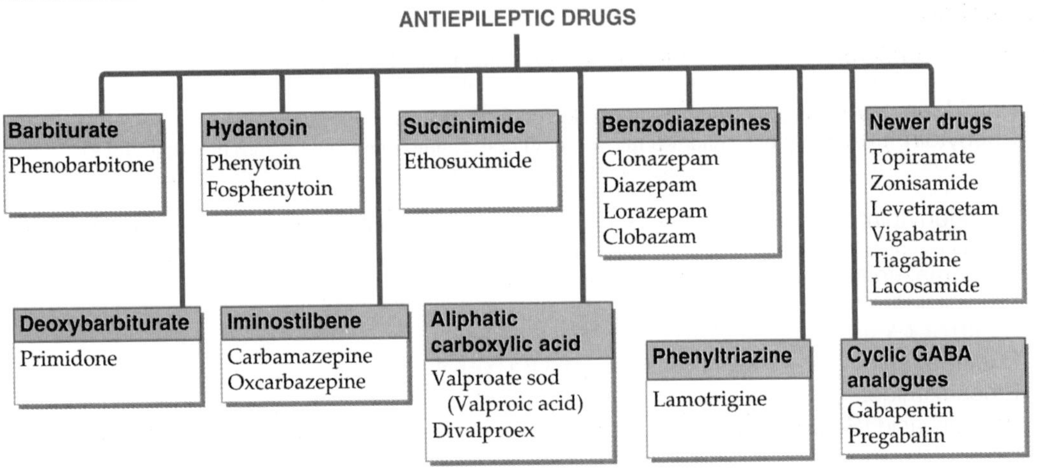
ANTIEPILEPTIC DRUGS
Barbiturate
Phenobarbitone
Hydantoin
Phenytoin
Fosphenytoin
Succinimide
Ethosuximide
Benzodiazepines
Clonazepam
Diazepam
Lorazepam
Clobazam
Newer drugs
Topiramate
Zonisamide
Levetiracetam
Vigabatrin
Tiagabine
Lacosamide
Deoxybarbiturate
Primidone
Iminostilbene
Carbamazepine
Oxcarbazepine
Aliphatic carboxylic acid
Valproate sod (Valproic acid)
Divalproex
Phenyltriazine
Lamotrigine
Cyclic GABA analogues
Gabapentin
Pregabalin

Preparations

1. **Phenobarbitone:** 60 mg OD–TDS (child 3–6 mg/kg/day), 100–200 mg i.m./i.v.; GARDENAL 30, 60 mg tab; LUMINAL 30 mg tab; PHENOBARBITONE SOD 200 mg/ml inj.
2. **Primidone:** 250–500 mg BD (child 10–20 mg/kg/day); MYSOLINE 250 mg tab.
3. **Phenytoin:** 100–200 mg BD (child 5–8 mg/kg/day) oral, 25 mg/min slow i.v. injection (max 1.0 g); DILANTIN 25 mg, 100 mg cap., 100 mg/4 ml oral suspension, 100 mg/2 ml inj.; EPTOIN 50, 100 mg tab, 25 mg/ml syr; FENTOIN-ER 100 mg extended release cap.
4. **Fosphenytoin:** 25-100 mg (as phenytoin sod. equivalent)/min i.v. injection (max 1.0 g) for generalized convulsive status epilepticus; FOSOLIN 50 mg/ml inj in 2 ml and 10 ml amp.
5. **Carbamazepine:** 200–400 mg TDS, children 15–30 mg/kg/day; TEGRETOL, MAZETOL 100, 200, 400 mg tab, 100 mg/5 ml syr; CARBATOL 100, 200, 400 mg tab; MAZETOL-SR, TEGRITAL-CR 200, 400 mg sustained release tabs.
6. **Oxcarbazepine:** 300–600 mg BD; OXCARB, OXEP, OXETOL 150, 300, 600 mg tabs.
7. **Ethosuximide:** 20–30 mg/kg/day; ZARONTIN 250 mg/5 ml syr.
8. **Valproic acid (Sodium valproate):** Adults—start with 200 mg TDS, maximum 800 mg TDS; children—15–30 mg/kg/day; VALPARIN CHRONO 200, 300, 500 mg tabs, 200 mg/5 ml syr, ENCORATE 200, 300, 500 mg regular tabs and controlled release tabs, 200 mg/5 ml syr, 100 mg/ml inj.
9. **Divalproex:** Epilepsy—initially 15 mg/kg/day, increase gradually as required (max 60 mg/kg/day);
   Bipolar disorder—250–500 mg TDS;
   Migraine 250–500 mg BD; DIPROEX, VALANCE, DEPAKOTE 125, 250, 500 mg tabs.
10. **Clonazepam:** Adults 0.5–5 mg TDS, children 0.02–0.2 mg/kg/day; status epilepticus 1–2 mg slow i.v. inj; LONAZEP, CLONAPAX, RIVOTRIL 0.5, 1.0, 2.0 mg tab.

11. **Diazepam:** for status epilepticus—10 mg (0.2–0.3 mg/kg) slow i.v. injection (2 mg/min), repeat fractional doses as required (max 100 mg/day); for febrile convulsions 0.5 mg/kg rectal instillation, repeat 12 hourly for 48 hours; VALIUM, CALMPOSE, PLACIDOX 10 mg/2 ml inj.
12. **Lorazepam:** for status epilepticus—4 mg (0.1 mg/kg in children) slow i.v. injection (2 mg/min); CALMESE 4 mg/2 ml inj.
13. **Clobazam:** start with 10–20 mg at bed time, can be increased upto 60 mg/day; FRISIUM, LOBAZAM, CLOZAM 5, 10, 20 mg cap.
14. **Lamotrigine:** 50 mg/day initially, increase upto 300 mg/day as needed. LAMITOR, LAMETEC, LAMIDUS 25, 50, 100 mg tabs.
15. **Gabapentin:** start with 300 mg OD, increase to 300–600 mg TDS as required; NEURONTIN, GABANTIN 300 mg, 400 mg cap, GABAPIN 100, 300, 400 mg cap.
16. **Pregabalin:** 75–150 mg BD, max. 600/day (used primarily for neuropathic pain). PREEGA, NEUGABA, TRUGABA 75, 150 mg caps.
17. **Vigabatrin:** 2–4 g/day, child 40–100 mg/kg/day.
18. **Topiramate:** Initially 25 mg OD, increase weekly upto 100–200 mg BD as required, child 5–10 mg/kg/day. TOPEX, EPITOP, TOPAMATE, NEXTOP 25, 50, 100 mg tabs.
19. **Zonisamide:** 25–100 mg BD (not for children); ZONISEP, ZONICARE, ZONIT 50, 100 mg cap.
20. **Levetiracetam:** 0.5 g BD, increase upto 1.0 g BD; children 4–15 years 10–30 mg/kg/day. EPIFAST, TORLEVA, LEVROXA, LEVTAM 250, 500, 750 mg tabs.

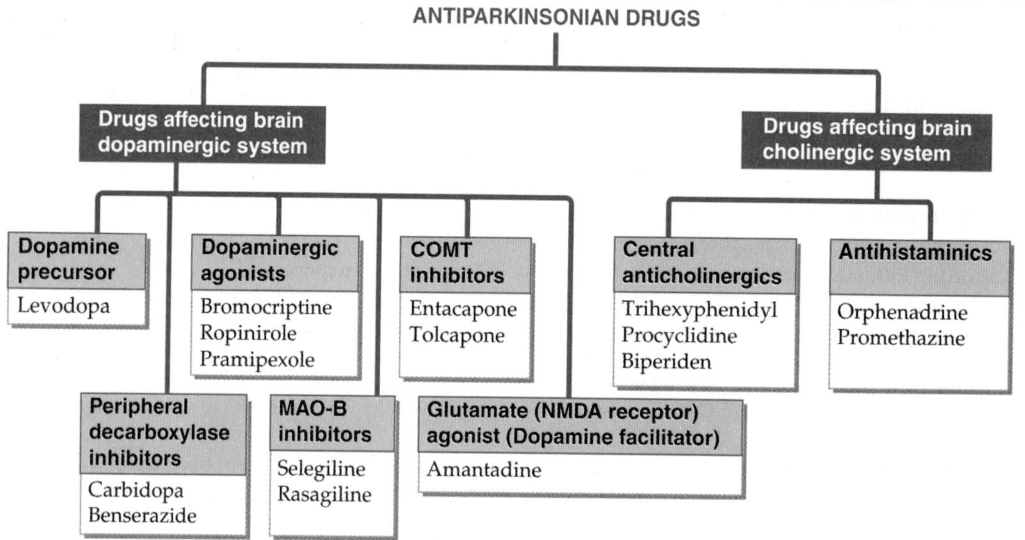
ANTIPARKINSONIAN DRUGS
Drugs affecting brain dopaminergic system
Drugs affecting brain cholinergic system
Dopamine precursor
Levodopa
Dopaminergic agonists
Bromocriptine
Ropinirole
Pramipexole
COMT inhibitors
Entacapone
Tolcapone
Central anticholinergics
Trihexyphenidyl
Procyclidine
Biperiden
Antihistaminics
Orphenadrine
Promethazine
Peripheral decarboxylase inhibitors
Carbidopa
Benserazide
MAO-B inhibitors
Selegiline
Rasagiline
Glutamate (NMDA receptor) agonist (Dopamine facilitator)
Amantadine

Preparations

1. **Levodopa:** Start with 0.25 g BD after meals, gradually increase till adequate response is obtained. Usual dose is 2–3 g/day. LEVOPA, BIDOPAL 0.5 g tab.

2. **Carbidopa/Benserazide + Levodopa combination:** Usual daily maintenance dose of levodopa is 0.4–0.8 g along with 75–100 mg carbidopa or 100–200 mg benserazide, given in 3–4 divided doses. Therapy is started at a low dose and suitable preparations are chosen according to the needs of individual patients, increasing the dose as required.

	Carbidopa (per tab/cap)		*Levodopa*
TIDOMET-LS, SYNDOPA-110,	10 mg	+	100 mg
SINEMET, DUODOPA-110	10 mg	+	100 mg
TIDOMET PLUS, SYNDOPA PLUS	25 mg	+	100 mg
TIDOMET FORTE, SYNDOPA-275	25 mg	+	250 mg

BENSPAR, MADOPAR: Benserazide 25 mg + levodopa 100 mg cap.

3. **Bromocriptine:** Start with 1.25 mg once at night, increase gradually as needed upto 5–10 mg TDS, as supplement to carbidopa-levodopa combination.
PROCTINAL, PARLODEL, SICRIPTIN 1.25 mg, 2.5 mg tabs, ENCRIPT 2.5, 5 mg tabs.

4. **Ropinirole:** Starting dose is 0.25 mg TDS, titrated to a maximum of 4–8 mg TDS. Early cases generally require 1–2 mg TDS.
ROPITOR, ROPARK, ROPEWAY 0.25, 0.5, 1.0, 2.0 mg tabs; also 1, 2, 4 and 8 mg ER tabs.

5. **Pramipexole:** Starting dose 0.125 mg TDS, titrate to 0.5–1.5 mg TDS; PRAMIPEX 0.5 mg tab., PARPEX 0.5, 1.0, 1.5 mg tabs, PRAMIROL 0.125, 0.25, 0.5, 1.0, 1.5 mg tabs.
6. **Selegiline:** 5 mg with breakfast and with lunch, either alone (in early cases) or with levodopa. Reduce by 1/4th levodopa dose after 2–3 days of adding selegiline. ELDEPRYL 5, 10 mg tab, SELERIN, SELGIN 5 mg tab.
7. **Rasagiline:** 1 mg OD in the morning; RELGIN, RASALECT 0.5, 1.0 mg tabs; RASIPAR 1.0 mg tab.
8. **Entacapone:** 200 mg with each dose of levodopa-carbidopa (max 1600 mg/day); ADCAPON 100 mg tab, COMTAN 200 mg tab.
9. **Amantidine:** 100 mg BD. AMANTREL, COMANTREL 200 mg tab.
10. **Trihexyphenidyl (benzhexol):** 2–10 mg/day. PACITANE, PARBENZ 2 mg tab.
11. **Procyclidine:** 5–20 mg/day; KEMADRIN 2.5, 5 mg tab.
12. **Biperiden:** 2–10 mg/day oral, i.m. or i.v.: DYSKINON 2 mg tab., 5 mg/ml inj.
13. **Orphenadrine:** 100–300 mg/day; DISIPAL, ORPHIPAL 50 mg tab.
14. **Promethazine:** 25–75 mg/day; PHENERGAN 10, 25 mg tab.

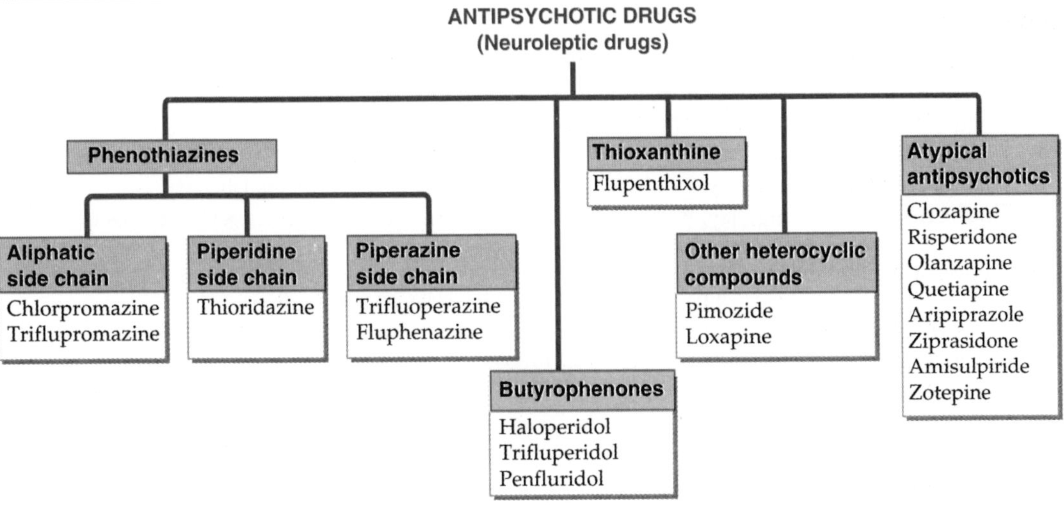
ANTIPSYCHOTIC DRUGS
(Neuroleptic drugs)
Phenothiazines
Aliphatic side chain
Chlorpromazine
Triflupromazine
Piperidine side chain
Thioridazine
Piperazine side chain
Trifluoperazine
Fluphenazine
Butyrophenones
Haloperidol
Trifluperidol
Penfluridol
Thioxanthine
Flupenthixol
Other heterocyclic compounds
Pimozide
Loxapine
Atypical antipsychotics
Clozapine
Risperidone
Olanzapine
Quetiapine
Aripiprazole
Ziprasidone
Amisulpiride
Zotepine

Preparations

1. **Chlorpromazine:** 100–800 mg/day; CHLORPROMAZINE, LARGACTIL 10, 25, 50, 100 mg tab. 5 mg/5 ml (pediatric) & 25 mg/5 ml (adult) syr., 50 mg/2 ml inj.
2. **Triflupromazine:** 50–200 mg/day; SIQUIL 10 mg tab; 10 mg/ml inj.
3. **Thioridazine:** 100–400 mg/day; MELLERIL 25, 100 mg tab, THIORIL 10, 25, 50 mg tab.
4. **Trifluoperazine:** 2–20 mg/day; TRINICALM 1, 5 mg tab, NEOCALM 5, 10 mg tab.
5. **Fluphenazine:** 1–10 mg/day; ANATENSOL 1 mg tab, 0.5 mg/ml elixir; ANATENSOL DECANOATE 25 mg/ml (as decanoate) for i.m. injection, 1–2 ml every 2–4 weeks.
6. **Haloperidol:** 2–20 mg/day; SERENACE 1.5, 5, 10, 20 mg tab; 2 mg/ml liq, 5 mg/ml inj., SENORM 1.5, 5, 10 mg tab, 5 mg/ml inj., HALOPIDOL 2, 20 mg tab, 2 mg/ml liq, 10 mg/ml drops.
7. **Trifluperidol:** 1–8 mg/day; TRIPERIDOL 0.5 mg tab, 2.5 mg/ml inj.
8. **Penfluridol:** 20–60 mg (max. 120 mg) once weekly; SEMAP, FLUMAP, PENFLUR 20 mg tab.
9. **Flupenthixol:** 3–15 mg/day; FLUANXOL 0.5, 1, 3 mg tab; FLUANXOL DEPOT 20 mg/ml in 1 and 2 ml amp.
10. **Pimozide:** 2–6 mg/day; ORAP, NEURAP, PIMODAC 2, 4 mg tab.
11. **Loxapine:** 20–50 mg/day; LOXAPAC 10, 25, 50 mg caps, 25 mg/ 5 ml liquid.
12. **Clozapine:** 100–300 mg/day; LOZAPIN, SIZOPIN, SKIZORIL 25, 100 mg tabs.
13. **Risperidone:** 2–8 mg/day; RESPIDON, SIZODON, RISPERDAL 1, 2, 3, 4 mg tabs.
14. **Olanzapine:** 2.5–20 mg/day; OLACE, OLANDUS 2.5, 5, 7.5, 10 mg tabs, OLZAP 5, 10 mg tab.
15. **Quetiapine:** 50–400 mg/day; QUEL, SOCALM, SEROQUIN 25, 100, 200 mg tabs.
16. **Aripiprazole:** 10–30 mg/day; ARIPRA, ARILAN, BILIEF 10, 15 mg tabs, ARIVE 10, 15, 20, 30 mg tabs.

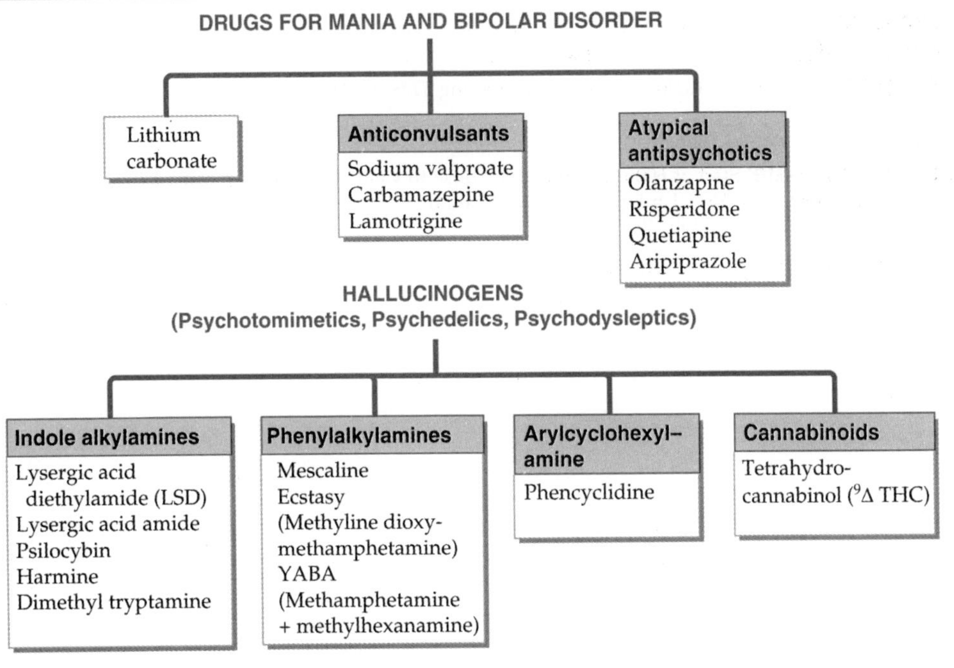
DRUGS FOR MANIA AND BIPOLAR DISORDER
Lithium carbonate
Anticonvulsants
Sodium valproate
Carbamazepine
Lamotrigine
Atypical antipsychotics
Olanzapine
Risperidone
Quetiapine
Aripiprazole
HALLUCINOGENS
(Psychotomimetics, Psychedelics, Psychodysleptics)
Indole alkylamines
Lysergic acid diethylamide (LSD)
Lysergic acid amide
Psilocybin
Harmine
Dimethyl tryptamine
Phenylalkylamines
Mescaline
Ecstasy
(Methyline dioxy-methamphetamine)
YABA
(Methamphetamine + methylhexanamine)
Arylcyclohexyl–amine
Phencyclidine
Cannabinoids
Tetrahydro-cannabinol (⁹Δ THC)

17. **Ziprasidone:** 80–160 mg/day; AZONA, ZIPSYDON 20, 40, 80 mg tabs.
18. **Amisulpiride:** 50–300 mg/day in 2 doses; SULPITAC, AMIPRIDE, ZONAPRIDE 50, 100, 200 mg tabs.
19. **Zotepine:** 25 mg TDS initially, increase upto 100 mg TDS; ZOLEPTIL, NIPOLEPT 25, 50 mg tabs.

Drugs for Mania and Bipolar Disorder

1. **Lithium carbonate:** Start at 600 mg/day, adjust dose to yield steady-state plasma level of 0.5–0.8 mEq/L (for bipolar disorder) or 0.8–1.1 mEq/L (for acute mania);
   LICAB, LITHOSUN 300 mg tab, 400 mg SR tab.

Note: *See* Index for preparations of other drugs.

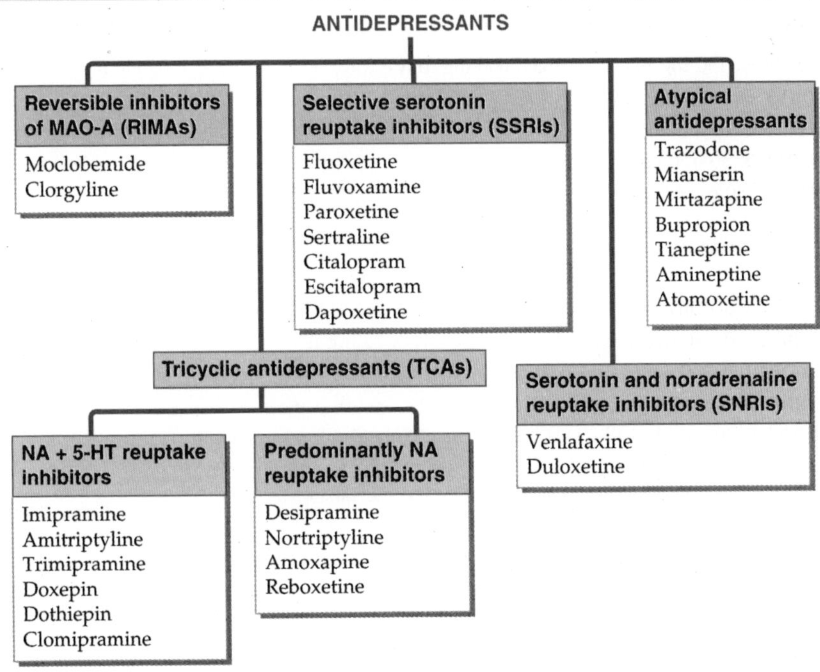
ANTIDEPRESSANTS
Reversible inhibitors of MAO-A (RIMAs)
Moclobemide
Clorgyline
Selective serotonin reuptake inhibitors (SSRIs)
Fluoxetine
Fluvoxamine
Paroxetine
Sertraline
Citalopram
Escitalopram
Dapoxetine
Atypical antidepressants
Trazodone
Mianserin
Mirtazapine
Bupropion
Tianeptine
Amineptine
Atomoxetine
Tricyclic antidepressants (TCAs)
Serotonin and noradrenaline reuptake inhibitors (SNRIs)
Venlafaxine
Duloxetine
NA + 5-HT reuptake inhibitors
Imipramine
Amitriptyline
Trimipramine
Doxepin
Dothiepin
Clomipramine
Predominantly NA reuptake inhibitors
Desipramine
Nortriptyline
Amoxapine
Reboxetine

Preparations

1. **Moclobemide:** 150 mg BD–TDS (max. 600 mg/day); RIMAREX, TRIMA 150, 300 mg tabs.
2. **Imipramine:** 50–200 mg/day; DEPSONIL, ANTIDEP 25 mg tab, 75 mg SR cap.
3. **Amitriptyline:** 50–200 mg/day; AMLINE, SAROTENA, TRYPTOMER, 10, 25, 75 mg tabs.
4. **Trimipramine:** 50–150 mg/day; SURMONTIL 10, 25 mg tab.
5. **Doxepin:** 50–150 mg/day; SPECTRA, DOXIN, DOXETAR 10, 25, 75 mg tab/cap; NOCTADERM 5% cream (to relieve itching).
6. **Clomipramine:** 50–150 mg/day; CLOFRANIL 10, 25, 50 mg tab, 75 mg SR tab, CLONIL, ANAFRANIL 10, 25 mg tab;
7. **Dothiepin (Dosulpin):** 50–150 mg/day; PROTHIADEN, DOTHIN 25, 75 mg tab.
8. **Nortriptyline:** 50–150 mg/day; SENSIVAL, PRIMOX 25 mg tab.
9. **Amoxapine:** 100–300 mg/day; DEMOLOX 50, 100 mg tab.
10. **Reboxetine:** 4–8 mg/day; NAREBOX 4, 8 mg tabs.
11. **Fluoxetine:** 20–40 mg/day; FLUDAC 20 mg cap, 20 mg/5 ml susp; FLUNIL 10, 20 mg caps; FLUPAR, PRODAC 20 mg cap.
12. **Fluvoxamine:** 50–200 mg/day; FLUVOXIN 50, 100 mg tab.
13. **Paroxetine:** 20–50 mg/day; XET 10, 20, 30, 40 mg tabs.
14. **Sertraline:** 50–150 mg/day; SERENATA, SERLIN, SERTIL 50, 100 mg tabs.
15. **Citalopram:** 20–40 mg/day; CELICA 10, 20, 40 mg tabs.
16. **Escitalopram:** 10–20 mg OD; ESDEP, FELIZ-S 5, 10, 20 mg tabs.
17. **Dapoxetine:** 60 mg 1 hour before intercourse, elderly 30 mg; SUSTINEX, DURALAST, KUTUB 30, 60 mg tabs.

18. **Trazodone:** 50–200 mg/day; TRAZODAC 25, 50 mg tab, TRAZONIL, TRAZALON 25, 50, 100 mg tabs.
19. **Mianserin:** 30–100 mg/day; TETRADEP 10, 20, 30 mg tab, SERIDAC 10, 30 mg tab.
20. **Bupropion:** 150–300 mg/day; SMOQUIT–SR, BUPRON–SR 150 mg tab.
21. **Mirtazapine:** 15–45 mg/day; MIRT 15, 30, 45 mg tabs, MIRTAZ 15, 30 mg tab.
22. **Venlafaxine:** 75–150 mg/day; VENLOR 25, 37.5, 75 mg tabs, VENIZ-XR 37.5, 75, 150 mg ER caps.
23. **Tianeptine:** 12.5 mg BD–TDS; STABLON 12.5 mg tab.
24. **Amineptine:** 100 mg BD at breakfast and lunch; SURVECTOR 100 mg tab.
25. **Duloxetine:** 30–80 mg/day; DELOK, DULANE, DUZAC 20, 30, 40 mg caps.

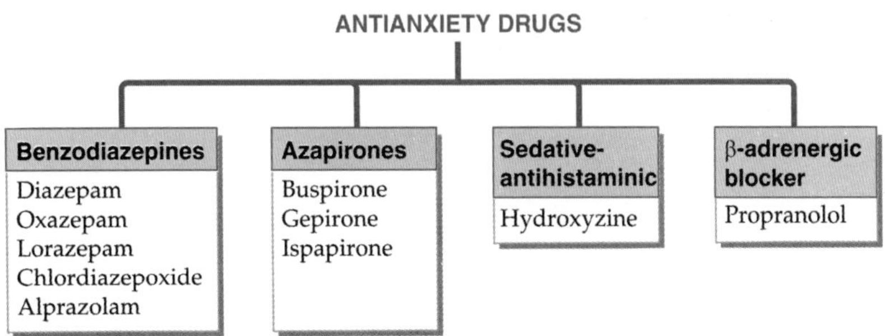

Preparations

1. **Diazepam:** 5–30 mg/day in 2–3 divided doses; VALIUM, PLACIDOX 2, 5, 10 mg tabs; CALMPOSE 5, 10 mg tab, 2 mg/5 ml syr.
2. **Chlordiazepoxide:** 20–100 mg/day in 2–3 divided doses, LIBRIUM 10, 25 mg tabs; EQUILIBRIUM 10 mg tab.
3. **Oxazepam:** 30–60 mg/day in 2–3 divided doses; SEREPAX 15, 30 mg tabs.
4. **Lorazepam:** 1–6 mg/day in 1–2 divided doses; LARPOSE, ATIVAN 1, 2 mg tab. CALMESE 1, 2 mg tabs, 4 mg/2 ml inj.
5. **Alprazolam:** 0.25–1.0 mg TDS; upto 6 mg/day in panic disorder; ALPRAX 0.25, 0.5, 1.0 mg tabs., 0.5, 1.0, 1.5 mg SR tabs; ALZOLAM 0.25, 0.5, 1.0 mg tabs; 1.5 mg SR tab, ALPROCONTIN 0.5, 1.0, 1.5 mg CR tabs. RESTYL-SR 0.5, 1.0, 1.5 mg SR tabs.
6. **Buspirone:** 5–15 mg 1–3 times daily; BUSCALM, ANXIPAR, BUSPIN 5, 10 mg tabs.
7. **Hydroxyzine:** 50–200 mg/day; ATARAX 10, 25 mg tabs, 10 mg/5 ml syr, 25 mg/2 ml inj.

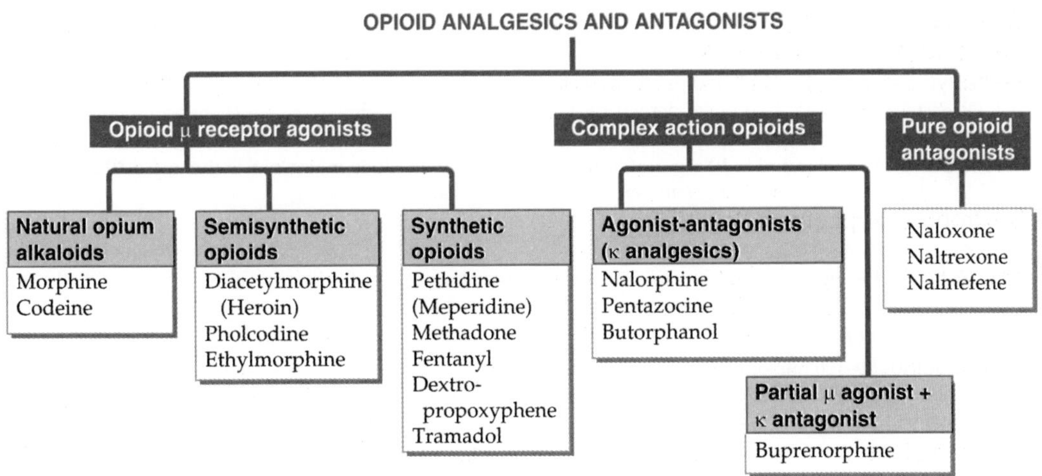

Preparations

Opioid Analgesics

1. **Morphine:** 10–50 mg oral, 10–15 mg i.m. or s.c., 2–6 mg i.v.; 2–3 mg epidural/intrathecal; children 0.1–0.2 mg/kg i.m. or s.c. MORPHINE SULPHATE 10 mg/ml inj; MORCONTIN 10, 30, 60, 100 mg continuous release tabs; 30–100 mg BD; RILIMORF 10, 20 mg tabs, 60 mg SR tab.

2. **Codeine:** 30–60 mg oral; CODEINE 15 mg tab, 15 mg/5 ml syr.
3. **Pethidine:** 50–100 mg oral/i.m./s.c., 10–15 mg i.v. (rarely); PETHIDINE 50, 100 mg tabs, 100 mg/2 ml inj.
4. **Fentanyl:** 2–4 μg/kg i.v.; 12.5–100 μg/hr transdermal; TROFENTYL, FENT 50 μg/ml in 2 ml amp and 10 ml vial, DUROGESIC transdermal patch delivering 12.5 μg/hr, 25 μg/hr, 50 μg/hr, 75 μg/hr and 100 μg per hour; the patch is changed every 3 days.
5. **Methadone:** As analgesic 2.5–10 mg oral/i.m. (not s.c.); for methadone maintenance therapy 5-40 mg per day; METHADONE 5 mg/ml and 10 mg/ml syr; 5, 10, 20, 40 mg tabs.
6. **Dextropropoxyphene:** 60–120 mg oral; PARVODEX 60 mg cap; PARVON, PROXYVON, WALAGESIC: dextropropoxyphene 65 mg + paracetamol 400 mg cap; WYGESIC, SUDHINOL 65 mg + paracetamol 650 mg cap.
7. **Tramadol:** 50–100 mg oral/i.m./slow i.v. infusion (children 1–2 mg/kg) 4–6 hourly. CONTRAMAL, DOMADOL, TRAMAZAC 50 mg cap, 100 mg SR tab; 50 mg/ml inj in 1 and 2 ml amps.

Opioid Agonist-Antagonists and Pure Antagonists

1. **Pentazocine:** 50–100 mg, oral, 30–60 mg i.m., s.c., FORTWIN 25 mg tab., 30 mg/ml inj., FORTSTAR, SUSEVIN 30 mg/ml inj; FORTAGESIC pentazocine 15 mg + paracetamol 500 mg tab.
2. **Butorphanol:** 1–4 mg i.m./i.v.; BUTRUM 1 mg/ml and 2 mg/ml inj.
3. **Buprenorphine:** 0.3–0.6 mg i.m., s.c. or slow i.v., also sublingual 0.2–0.4 mg 6–8 hourly; NORPHIN, TIDIGESIC 0.3 mg/ml inj. 1 and 2 ml amps. 0.2 mg sublingual tab; BUPRIGESIC, PENTOREL 0.3 mg/ml inj in 1, 2 ml amp.
4. **Naloxone:** Adults 0.4–0.8 mg i.v. every 2–3 min (max 10 mg); neonates 10 μg/kg in the umbilical cord; NARCOTAN 0.4 mg in 1 ml (adult) and 0.04 mg in 2 ml (infant) amps; NALOX, NEX 0.4 mg inj.
5. **Naltrexone:** 50 mg/day oral; NALTIMA, NALTROX 50 mg tab.

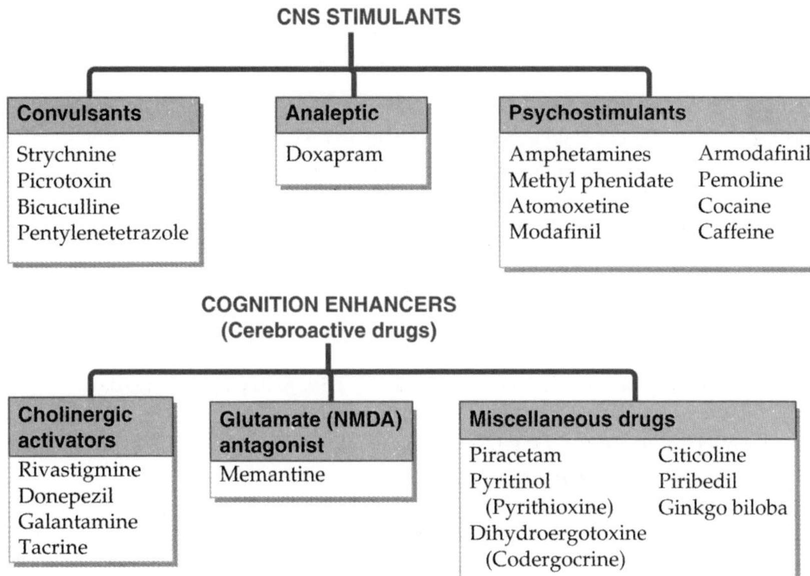
CNS STIMULANTS
Convulsants
Strychnine
Picrotoxin
Bicuculline
Pentylenetetrazole
Analeptic
Doxapram
Psychostimulants
Amphetamines
Methyl phenidate
Atomoxetine
Modafinil
Armodafinil
Pemoline
Cocaine
Caffeine
COGNITION ENHANCERS
(Cerebroactive drugs)
Cholinergic activators
Rivastigmine
Donepezil
Galantamine
Tacrine
Glutamate (NMDA) antagonist
Memantine
Miscellaneous drugs
Piracetam
Pyritinol
(Pyrithioxine)
Dihydroergotoxine
(Codergocrine)
Citicoline
Piribedil
Ginkgo biloba

Preparations

CNS Stimulants

1. **Doxapram:** 40–80 mg i.m. or i.v.; 0.5–2 mg/kg/hr i.v. infusion. CAROPRAM 20 mg/ml in 5 ml amp.
2. **Methylphenidate:** Adults 5–10 mg BD, child 0.25 mg/kg/day (max 1 mg/kg/day); RETALIN 5, 10, 20, 30 mg tab.
3. **Atomoxetine:** 0.5 mg/kg OD in the morning (max 1.2 mg/kg/day) in children; adults 40 mg OD (max. 100 mg OD). ATTENTROL 10, 18, 25, 40 mg caps; AXEPTA 18, 25 mg cap.
4. **Modafinil:** 100-200 mg morning and afternoon (for day time sleepiness), 200 mg 1 hour before starting night shift. MODALERT, PROVAKE 100, 200 mg tabs.
5. **Caffeine:** 20–100 mg oral; in CAFERGOT: Caffeine 100 mg + ergotamine 1 mg tab. MICROPYRIN: Caffeine 20 mg + aspirin 350 mg tab.

Cognition Enhancers

1. **Rivastigmine:** Start with 1.5 mg BD, increase every 2 weeks by 1.5 mg/day upto 6 mg/day; EXELON, RIVAMER 1.5, 3.0, 6.0 mg caps.
2. **Donepezil:** 5 mg once at bed time (max. 10 mg OD); DONECEPT, DOPEZIL, DORENT 5, 10 mg tabs.
3. **Galantamine:** 4 mg BD (max. 12 mg BD); GALAMER 4, 8, 12 mg tabs.
4. **Memantine:** 5 mg OD, increase up to 10 mg BD; ADMENTA, MENTADEM 5, 10 mg tabs, ALMANTIN 5 mg tab.
5. **Piracetam:** 0.8–1 g TDS; children 20 mg/kg BD–TDS; 1–3 g i.m. 6 hourly in stroke/head injury; NORMABRAIN, NEUROCETAM, NOOTROPIL 400, 800 mg cap, 500 mg/5 ml syr., 300 mg/ml inj.

6. **Pyritinol (Pyrithioxine):** 100–200 mg TDS, child 50–100 mg TDS oral, 200–400 mg 6 hourly (max. 1 g/day) i.v.; ENCEPHABOL 100, 200 mg tab, 100 mg/5 ml susp, 200 mg dry powder in vial with solvent for i.v. infusion.
7. **Dihydroergotoxine (Codergocrine):** 1–1.5 mg TDS oral/sublingual, 0.3 mg i.m. OD; HYDERGINE 1 mg tab, 0.3 mg/ml inj, CERELOID 1 mg tab.
8. **Piribedil:** 50 mg OD–BD; TRIVASTAL-LA 50 mg tab.
9. **Ginkgo biloba:** 40–80 mg TDS; GINKOCER, BILOVAS, GINKOBA 40 mg tab.
10. **Citicoline:** Oral 200–600 mg/day in divided doses;
    Parenteral 0.5–1.0 g/day i.m./i.v.
    STROLIN 500 mg tab, CITILIN, CITINOVA 500 mg tab, 500 mg/2 ml inj.

7 Cardiovascular Drugs

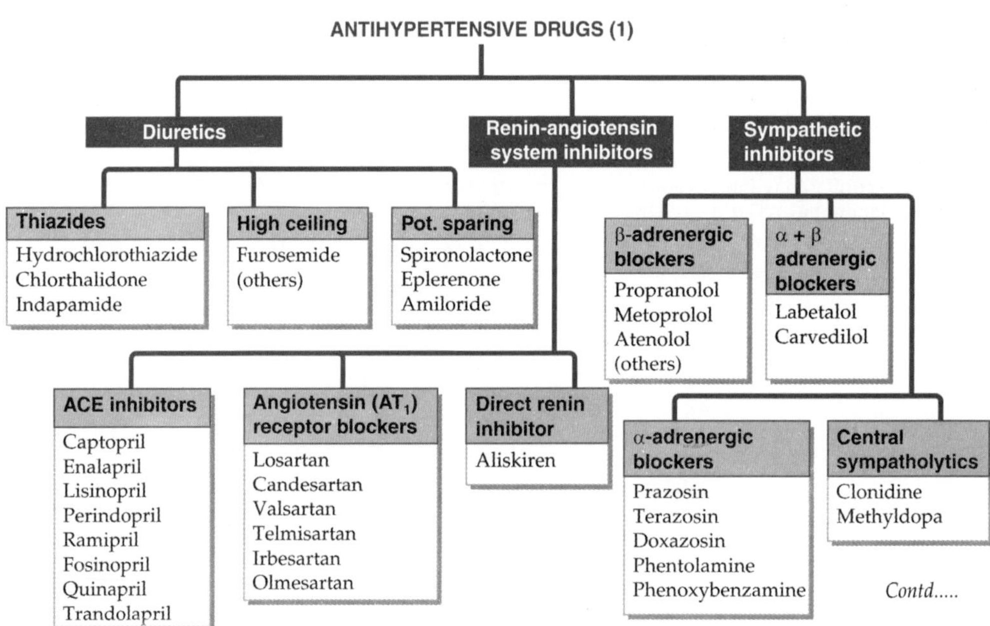

Contd.....

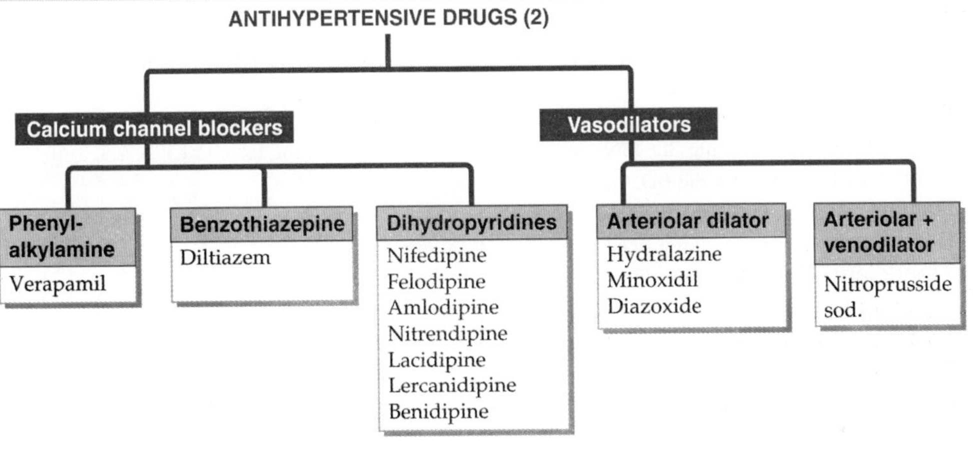
ANTIHYPERTENSIVE DRUGS (2)
Calcium channel blockers
Vasodilators
Phenyl-alkylamine
Verapamil
Benzothiazepine
Diltiazem
Dihydropyridines
Nifedipine
Felodipine
Amlodipine
Nitrendipine
Lacidipine
Lercanidipine
Benidipine
Arteriolar dilator
Hydralazine
Minoxidil
Diazoxide
Arteriolar + venodilator
Nitroprusside sod.

Preparations

1. **Captopril:** Initially 25 mg BD, increase upto 50 mg TDS as needed. To be taken 1 hr before or 2 hr after a meal; ANGIOPRIL 25 mg tab, ACETEN, CAPOTRIL 12.5, 25 mg tabs.
2. **Enalapril:** 2.5 mg OD–20 mg BD; ENAPRIL, ENVAS, ENAM 2.5, 5, 10, 20 mg tabs.
3. **Lisinopril:** 5 mg OD–20 mg BD; LINVAS, LISTRIL, LIPRIL 2.5, 5, 10 mg tabs, LISORIL 2.5, 5, 10, 20 mg tabs.
4. **Perindopril:** 2 mg OD–4 mg BD; COVERSYL 2, 4 mg tabs.
5. **Ramipril:** 1.25 mg OD–5 mg BD; CARDACE, RAMIRIL, CORPRIL, RPRIL 1.25, 2.5, 5 mg caps.
6. **Benazepril:** 10 mg OD–20 mg BD; BENACE 5, 10, 20 mg tabs.
7. **Trandolapril:** 2 mg OD–4 mg BD; ZETPRIL 1, 2 mg tabs.
8. **Fosinopril:** 10–40 mg OD; FOSINACE, FOVAS 10, 20 mg tabs.
9. **Imidapril:** Start with 5 mg (elderly 2.5 mg) OD, max. 10 mg BD; TANATRIL 5, 10 mg tabs.
10. **Quinapril:** 10–40 mg/day; ACCUPRIL-H Quinapril 20 mg + hydrochlorothiazide 12.5 mg tab.
11. **Losartan:** 50 mg OD (max. 50 mg BD), liver disease and volume depleted patients 25 mg OD; LOSAR, LOSACAR, TOZAR, ALSARTAN 25, 50 mg tabs.
12. **Candesartan:** 8 mg OD (max. 8 mg BD), liver/kidney disease patients 4 mg OD; CANDESAR 4, 8, 10 mg tabs, CANDILONG, CANDESTAN 4, 8 mg tabs.
13. **Irbesartan:** 150–300 mg OD; IROVEL, IRBEST 150, 300 mg tabs.
14. **Valsartan:** 80–160 mg OD; DIOVAN 40, 80, 160 mg tabs. STARVAL, VALZAAR 80, 160 mg tabs.
15. **Telmisartan:** 20–80 mg OD; TELMA, TELSAR, TELVAS 20, 40 mg tabs.
16. **Olmesartan medoxomil:** 20–40 mg OD; OLMAT 20, 40 mg tabs.
17. **Aliskiren:** 150–300 mg OD; RASILEZ 150 mg tab; RASILEZ-HC alongwith hydrochlorothiazide 12.5 mg.

18. **Verapamil:** 40–160 mg TDS oral, 5 mg by slow i.v. inj; CALAPTIN 40, 80 mg tab, 120, 240 mg SR tab; VPL 5 mg/2 ml inj, VASOPTEN 40, 80, 120 mg tabs.
19. **Diltiazem:** 30–60 mg TDS–QID oral; DILZEM 30, 60 mg tabs, 90 mg SR tab; 25 mg/5 ml inj; ANGIZEM 30, 60, 90, 120, 180 mg tab, DILTIME 30, 60 mg tab; 90, 120 mg SR tab.
20. **Nifedipine:** 5–20 mg BD–TDS oral; CALCIGARD, DEPIN, NIFELAT 5, 10 mg cap, also 10 mg, 20 mg SR (RETARD) tab., ADALAT RETARD 10, 20 mg SR tab.
21. **Felodipine:** 5–10 mg OD (max. 10 mg BD); FELOGARD, PLENDIL, RENDIL 2.5, 5, 10 mg ER tab.
22. **Amlodipine:** 5–10 mg OD; AMLOPRES, AMCARD, AMLOPIN, MYODURA 2.5, 5, 10 mg tabs.
23. **S(–) Amlodipine:** 2.5–5 mg OD; S-NUMLO 1.25, 2.5, 5.0 mg tabs; ESAM, S-AMCARD, ASOMEX 2.5, 5.0 mg tabs.
24. **Nitrendipine:** 5–20 mg OD (max. 20 mg BD); CARDIF, NITREPIN 10, 20 mg tab.
25. **Lacidipine:** 4–6 mg OD; LACIVAS, SINOPIL 2, 4 mg tabs.
26. **Benidipine:** 4–8 mg OD; CARITEC 4, 8 mg tabs.
27. **Lercanidipine:** 10–20 mg OD; LERKA, LEREZ 10, 20 mg tabs.
28. **Hydrochlorothiazide:** 12.5–50 mg OD; AQUAZIDE. HYDRAZIDE, HYDRIDE 12.5, 25, 50 mg tabs.
29. **Chlorthalidone:** 25–100 mg OD; HYTHALTON 100 mg tab.
30. **Indapamide:** 2.5 mg OD; LORVAS, NATRILIX 2.5 mg tab, NATRILIX-SR, DIURIX-SR 1.5 mg tab.
31. **Clonidine:** Start with 100 μg OD or BD, max 300 μg TDS, orally or i.m.; CATAPRES 150 μg tab, ARKAMIN 100 μg tab.
32. **Methyldopa:** 0.25–0.5 g BD–QID; EMDOPA, ALPHADOPA 250 mg tab.
33. **Hydralazine:** 25–50 mg OD–TDS; NEPRESOL 25 mg tab.
34. **Sodium nitroprusside:** Initiate i.v. infusion with 0.02 mg/min, titrate with lowering of blood pressure upto 0.1–0.3 mg/min; SONIDE, PRUSIDE, NIPRESS 50 mg in 5 ml inj.

Note: *See* Index for preparations of other drugs.

Some combined antihypertensive formulations

1. Amlodipine 5 mg + Lisinopril 5 mg—AMLOPRES-L, LISTRIL-AM
2. Amlodipine 5 mg + Atenolol 50 mg—AMCARD-AT, AMLOPIN-AT, AMLOPRES-AT
3. Amlodipine 5 mg + Enalapril 5 mg—AMACE, AMTAS-E
4. Atenolol 25 mg or 50 mg + Chlorthalidone 12.5 mg—TENOCLOR, TENORIC
5. Enalapril 10 mg + Hydrochlorothiazide 25 mg–ENACE-D, VASONORM-H
6. Ramipril 2.5 mg + Hydrochlorothiazide 12.5 mg—CARDACE-H
7. Losartan 50 mg + Hydrochlorothiazide 12.5 mg—LOSAR-H, TOZAAR-H, LOSACAR-H
8. Lisinopril 5 mg + Hydrochlorothiazide 12.5 mg—LISTRIL PLUS, LISORIL-HT
9. Losartan 50 mg + Ramipril 2.5 mg or 5 mg—TOZAAR-R, LAPIDO-R
10. Losartan 50 mg + Amlodipine 5 mg—AMCARD-LP, AMLOPRES-Z, LOSACAR-A
11. Losartan 50 mg + Ramipril 2.5 mg + Hydrochlorothiazide 12.5 mg—LOSANORM-HR
12. Irbesartan 150 mg + Hydrochlorothiazide 12.5 mg—IROVEL-H, XARB-H.

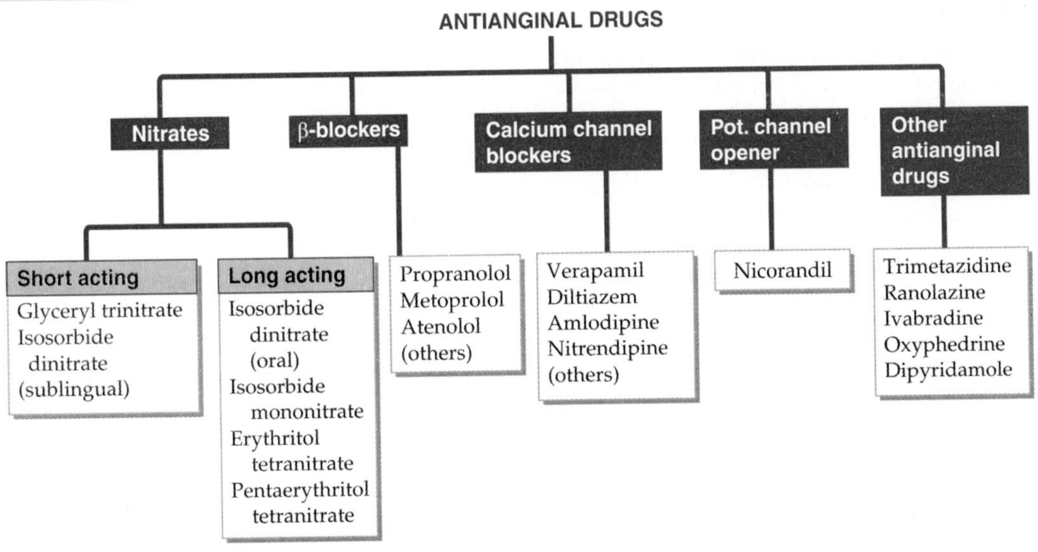
ANTIANGINAL DRUGS
Nitrates
β-blockers
Calcium channel blockers
Pot. channel opener
Other antianginal drugs
Short acting
Glyceryl trinitrate
Isosorbide dinitrate (sublingual)
Long acting
Isosorbide dinitrate (oral)
Isosorbide mononitrate
Erythritol tetranitrate
Pentaerythritol tetranitrate
Propranolol
Metoprolol
Atenolol
(others)
Verapamil
Diltiazem
Amlodipine
Nitrendipine
(others)
Nicorandil
Trimetazidine
Ranolazine
Ivabradine
Oxyphedrine
Dipyridamole

Preparations

1. **Glyceryl trinitrate (GTN), Nitroglycerine:**
   0.5 mg sublingual, 5–15 mg oral; ANGISED 0.5 mg tab, NITROLINGUAL spray, GTN spray 0.4 mg per spray; ANGISPAN-TR 2.5, 6.5 mg SR cap, NITROCONTIN, CORODIL 2.6, 6.4 mg CR tabs; One transdermal patch for 14–16 hr per day; NITRODERM-TTS 5 or 10 mg patch; 5–20 μg/min i.v.; MYOVIN, MILLISROL, NITROJECT 5 mg/ml inj.
2. **Isosorbide dinitrate:**
   5–10 mg sublingual; SORBITRATE 5, 10 mg tab; 10–20 mg oral; ISORDIL 5 mg sublingual & 10 mg oral tab; 20–40 mg sustained release oral; DITRATE 5, 10 mg tab; 20, 40 mg SR tab.
3. **Isosorbide-5-mononitrate:** 20–40 mg oral; MONOTRATE 10, 20, 40 mg tab, 50 mg SR tab, 5-MONO, MONOSORBITRATE 10, 20, 40 mg tab.
4. **Erythrityl tetranitrate:** 15–60 mg oral; CARDILATE 5, 15 mg tab.
5. **Pentaerythritol tetranitrate:** 10–40 mg oral; PERITRATE 10 mg tab; 80 mg sustained release oral; PERITRATE-SA 80 mg SR tab.
6. **Nicorandil: 5–20 mg BD;** NIKORAN, 5, 10 mg tabs, 2 mg/vial and 48 mg/multidose vial inj; KORANDIL 5, 10 mg tabs.
7. **Trimetazidine:** 20 mg TDS after meals; FLAVEDON, CARVIDON, TRIVEDON 20 mg tabs, 35 mg modified release tab.
8. **Ranolazine:** 0.5–1.0 g BD as SR tab; RANOZEX, REVULANT, RANX, CARTINEX, RANOLAZ 500 mg SR tab.
9. **Ivabradine:** 5–7.5 mg BD, elderly 2.5 mg BD; IVABRAD, BRADIA 5, 7.5 mg tab.
10. **Oxyphedrine:** 8–24 mg TDS oral, 4–8 mg i.v. OD–BD; ILDAMEN 8, 24 mg tab., 4 mg/2 ml inj.

Note: See Index for preparations of β-blockers and calcium channel blockers.

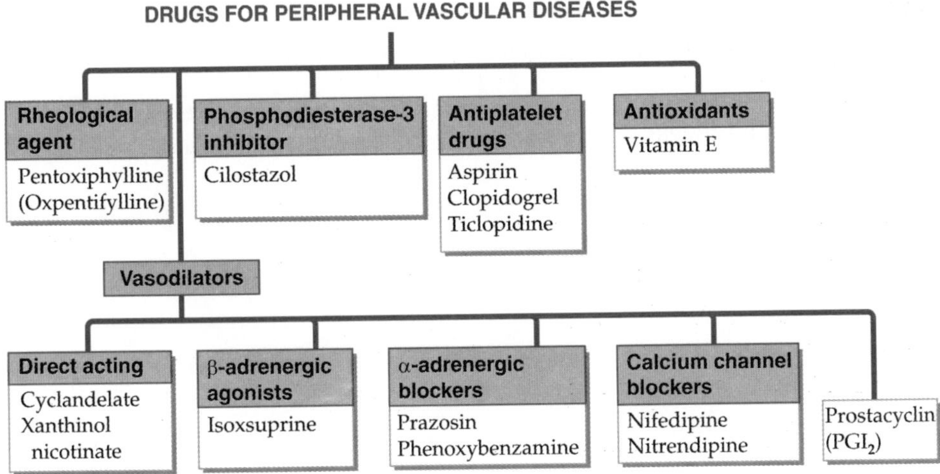
DRUGS FOR PERIPHERAL VASCULAR DISEASES
Rheological agent
Pentoxiphylline (Oxpentifylline)
Phosphodiesterase-3 inhibitor
Cilostazol
Antiplatelet drugs
Aspirin
Clopidogrel
Ticlopidine
Antioxidants
Vitamin E
Vasodilators
Direct acting
Cyclandelate
Xanthinol nicotinate
β-adrenergic agonists
Isoxsuprine
α-adrenergic blockers
Prazosin
Phenoxybenzamine
Calcium channel blockers
Nifedipine
Nitrendipine
Prostacyclin (PGI2)

Preparations

1. **Pentoxiphylline:** 400 mg BD–TDS; TRENTAL-400, FLEXITAL 400 mg SR tab, 300 mg/15 ml for slow i.v. injection.
2. **Cyclandelate:** 200–400 mg TDS; CYCLOSPASMOL, CYCLASYN 200, 400 mg tab/cap.
3. **Xanthinol nicotinate:** 300–600 mg TDS oral; 300 mg by i.m. or slow i.v. injection; COMPLAMINA 150 mg tab, 500 mg retard tab, 300 mg/2 ml inj.
4. **Cilostazol:** 100 mg BD half hour before or 2 hours after food; CILODOC, PLETOZ, STILOZ 50, 100 mg tabs.

Note: See Index for preparations of other drugs.

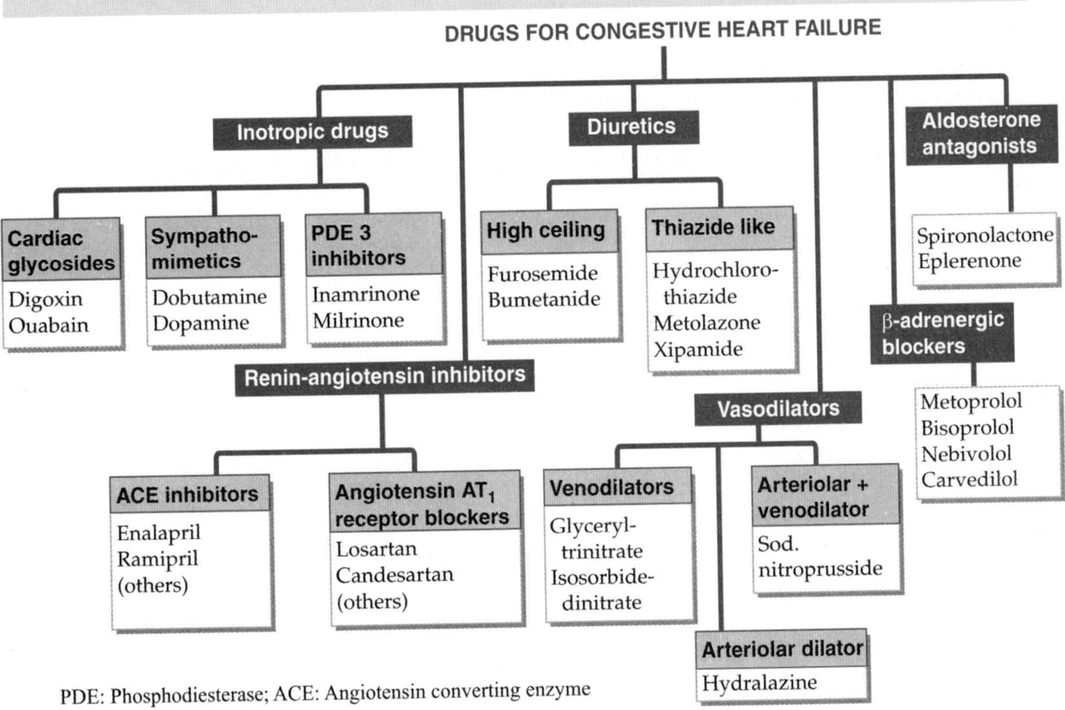

PDE: Phosphodiesterase; ACE: Angiotensin converting enzyme

Preparations

1. **Digoxin:** 0.25–0.5 mg/day (elderly 0.125–0.25 mg/day) oral adjusted according to response, 0.25 mg slow i.v. injection followed by 0.1 mg 1–2 hourly as needed; DIGOXIN 0.25 mg tab, 0.05 mg/ml pediatric elixir, 0.5 mg/2 ml inj. LANOXIN 0.25 mg tab, CARDIOXIN, DIXIN 0.25 mg tab, 0.5 mg/2 ml inj.
2. **Inamrinone (Amrinone):** 0.5 mg/kg i.v. bolus injection followed by 5–10 µg/kg/min i.v. infusion (max. 10 mg/kg in 24 hours). AMICOR, CARDIOTONE 5 mg/ml (as lactate) 20 ml amp.
3. **Milrinone:** 50 µg/kg i.v. bolus followed by 0.4–1.0 µg/kg/min infusion; PRIMACOR IV 10 mg/10 ml inj.

Note: See Index for preparations of other drugs.

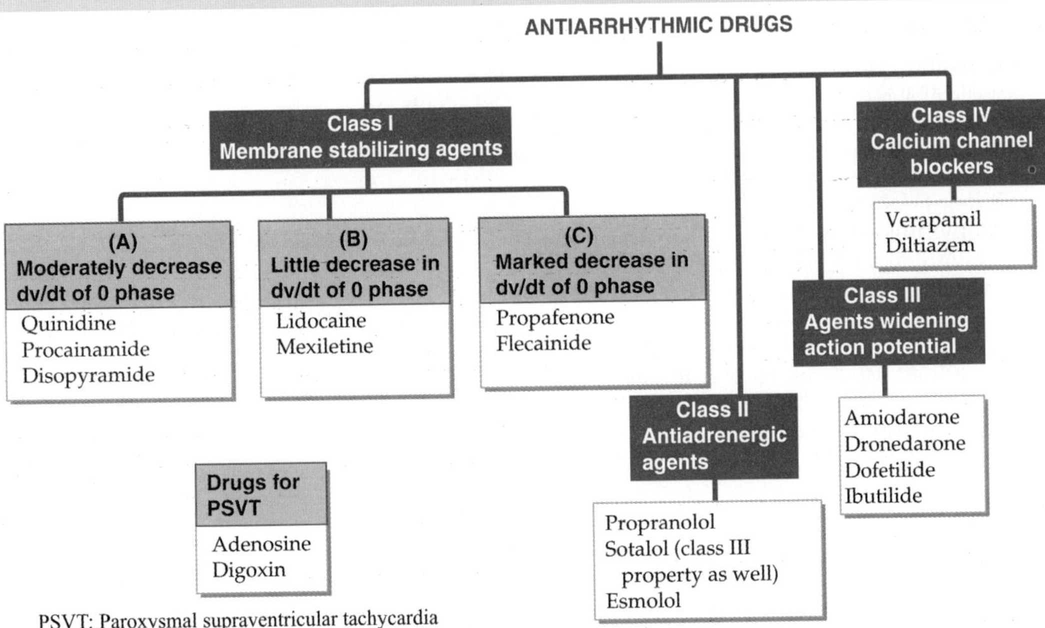

PSVT: Paroxysmal supraventricular tachycardia

Preparations

1. **Quinidine:** 100–200 mg TDS oral: rarely 100–300 mg slow i.v. inj. QUINIDINE SULPHATE 200 mg tab; QUININGA 300 mg tab, 600 mg/2 ml inj, NATCARDINE 100 mg tab.
2. **Procainamide:** for abolition of arrhythmia—0.5–1 g oral or i.m. followed by 0.25–0.5 g every 2 hours; or 500 mg i.v. loading dose (25 mg/min injection) followed by 2mg/kg/hour.
   Maintenance dose—0.5 g every 4–6 hours;
   PRONESTYL 250 mg tab., 1 g/10 ml inj.
3. **Disopyramide:** 100–150 mg 6 hourly oral; rarely 2 mg/kg by slow i.v. injection;
   NORPACE, 100, 150 mg cap, REGUBEAT 100 mg tab.
4. **Lidocaine (Lignocaine):** 50–100 mg bolus followed by 20–40 mg every 10–20 min or 1–3 mg/min infusion; XYLOCARD, GESICARD 20 mg/ml inj. (5, 50 ml vials). These preparations for cardiac use contain no preservative. The local anaesthetic preparations should not be used for this purpose.
5. **Mexiletine:** 100–250 mg i.v. over 10 min, 1 mg/min i.v. infusion. Oral: 150–200 mg TDS with meals;
   MEXITIL 50, 150 mg caps, 250 mg/10 ml inj.
6. **Propafenone:** 150 mg BD–300 mg TDS oral; RHYTHMONORM 150 mg tab.
7. **Propranolol:** 1 mg/min (max 5 mg) i.v. injection under close monitoring; 40–80 mg (max 160 mg) BD to QID oral; INDERAL, CIPLAR 10, 40, 80 mg tabs, 1 mg/ml inj, BETABLOCK 10, 40 mg tabs.
8. **Sotalol:** 40–80 mg BD–QID oral; SOTAGARD 40, 80 mg tabs.
9. **Esmolol:** 0.5 mg/kg in 1 min followed by 0.05–0.2 mg/kg/min i.v. infusion;
   MINIBLOCK 100 mg/10 ml, 250 mg/10 ml inj.
10. **Amiodarone:** 400–600 mg/day orally for few weeks, followed by 100–200 mg OD for maintenance; 100–300 mg (5 mg/kg) slow i.v. injection over 30–60 min;
    CORDARONE, ALDARONE, EURYTHMIC 100, 200 mg tabs, 150 mg/3 ml inj.

11. **Verapamil:** 5 mg slow i.v. injection over 2–3 min (to terminate PSVT), 60–120 mg TDS orally for maintenance and to control ventricular rate in atrial fibrillation or flutter;
CALAPTIN 40, 80 mg tab; 120, 240 mg SR tab, 5 mg/2 ml inj.
12. **Diltiazem:** 25 mg by slow i.v. inj (to terminate PSVT and to rapidly control ventricular rate in atrial fibrillation or flutter), 30–60 mg TDS orally for maintenance;
DILZEM 30, 60 mg tabs, 90 mg SR tab; 25 mg/5 ml inj.
13. **Adenosine:** 6–12 mg (free base) by rapid i.v. injection in a central vein;
ADENOJECT, ADENOCOR, 3 mg adenosine base per ml in 2 ml and 10 ml amp.

8 Drugs Acting on Kidney

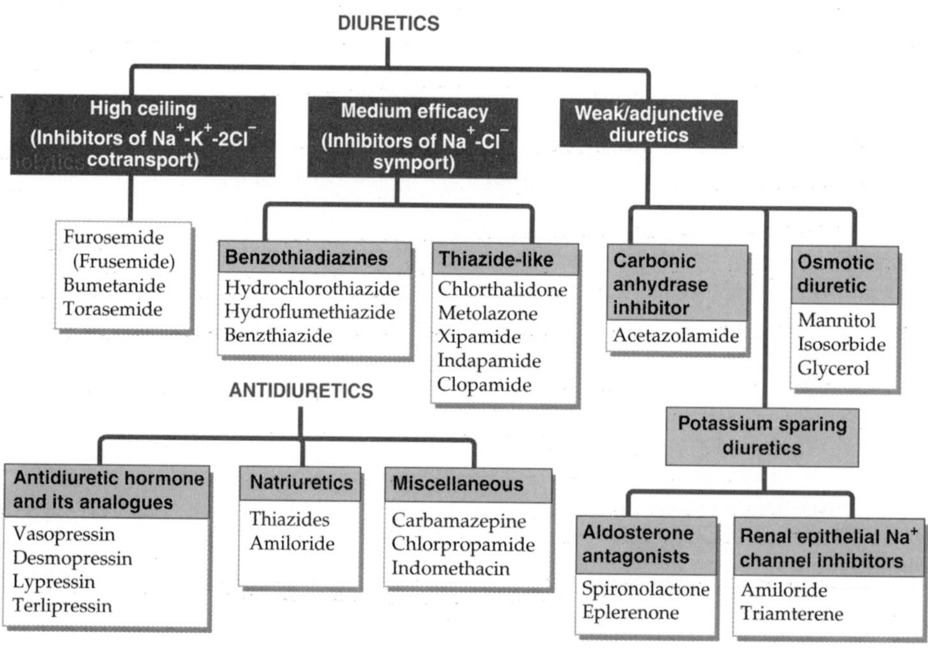

Preparations

Diuretics

1. **Furosemide (Frusemide):** Usually 20–80 mg once daily in the morning. In renal insufficiency, upto 200 mg 6 hourly given by i.m./i.v. route. In pulmonary edema 40–80 mg i.v.;
LASIX 40 mg tab., 20 mg/2 ml inj. LASIX HIGH DOSE 500 mg tab, 250 mg/25 ml inj; (solution degrades spontaneously on exposure to light), SALINEX 40 mg tab, FRUSENEX 40, 100 mg tab.
2. **Bumetanide:** 1–5 mg oral once daily in the morning, 2–4 mg i.v./i.m. (max 15 mg/day in renal failure);
BUMET 1 mg tab, 0.25 mg/ml inj.
3. **Torasemide:** 2.5–20 mg once daily in the morning;
DIURETOR 10, 20 mg tabs, DYTOR, TIDE 5, 10, 20, 100 mg tabs.
4. **Hydrochlorothiazide:** 12.5–100 mg OD in the morning; AQUAZIDE, THIAZIDE, HYDRIDE 12.5, 25, 50 mg tabs, ESIDREX 50 mg tab.
5. **Chlorthalidone:** 50–100 mg OD in the morning;
HYTHALTON 50, 100 mg tab, HYDRAZIDE, THALIZIDE 12.5, 25 mg tabs.
6. **Metolazone:** 5–20 mg OD in the morning; XAROXOLYN 5, 10 mg tab, DIUREM, METORAL 2.5, 5, 10 mg tabs.
7. **Xipamide:** 20–40 mg OD in the morning; XIPAMID 20 mg tab.
8. **Indapamide:** 2.5–5 mg OD in the morning; LORVAS 2.5 mg tab.
9. **Clopamide:** 10–60 mg OD in the morning; BRINALDIX 20 mg tab.
10. **Acetazolamide:** 250 mg OD–BD; DIAMOX, SYNOMAX 250 mg tab. IOPAR-SR 250 mg SR cap.
11. **Spironolactone:** 25–50 mg BD–QID; ALDACTONE 25, 50, 100 mg tabs; ALDACTIDE: Spironolactone 25 mg + hydroflumethiazide 25 mg tab; LACILACTONE, SPIROMIDE, Spironolactone 50 mg + furosemide 20 mg tab. TORLACTONE spironolactone 50 mg + torasemide 10 mg tab.

12. **Eplerenone:** 25–50 mg BD; EPTUS, EPLERAN, ALRISTA 25, 50 mg tabs.
13. **Triamterene:** 50–100 mg daily; DITIDE, triamterene 50 mg + benzthiazide 25 mg tab; FRUSEMENE, triamterene 50 mg + furosemide 20 mg tab.
14. **Amiloride:** 5–10 mg OD–BD; BIDURET, KSPAR Amiloride 5 mg + hydrochlorothiazide 50 mg tab, LASIRIDE, AMIFRU amiloride 5 mg + furosemide 40 mg tab.
15. **Mannitol:** 100–500 ml of 10–20% solution infused i.v.; MANNITOL 10%, 20% in 100, 350 and 500 ml vac.

Antidiuretics

1. **Aqueous Vasopressin (Arginine Vasopressin, AVP):** 5–10 U i.v/i.m./s.c.; PROSTACTON 10 U inj.
2. **Lypressin:** 10 IU i.m. or s.c. or 20 IU diluted in 100–200 ml of dextrose solution and infused i.v. over 10–20 min; PETRESIN, VASOPIN 20 IU/ml inj.
3. **Terlipressin:** 2 mg i.v., repeat 1–2 mg every 4–6 hours as needed;
   GLYPRESSIN, TERLINIS, T-PRESSIN 1 mg freez dried powder with 5 ml diluent for inj.
4. **Desmopressin (dDAVP):** *Intranasal:* Adults 10–40 μg/day in 2–3 divided doses, children 5–10 μg at bed time
   Oral: 0.1–0.2 mg TDS
   Parenteral (s.c. or i.v.) 2–4 μg/day in 2–3 divided doses.
   MINIRIN 100 μg/ml nasal spray (10 μg per actuation); 100 μg/ml intranasal solution in 2.5 ml bottle with applicator; 0.1 mg tablets; 4 μg/ml inj.

9 Drugs Affecting Blood

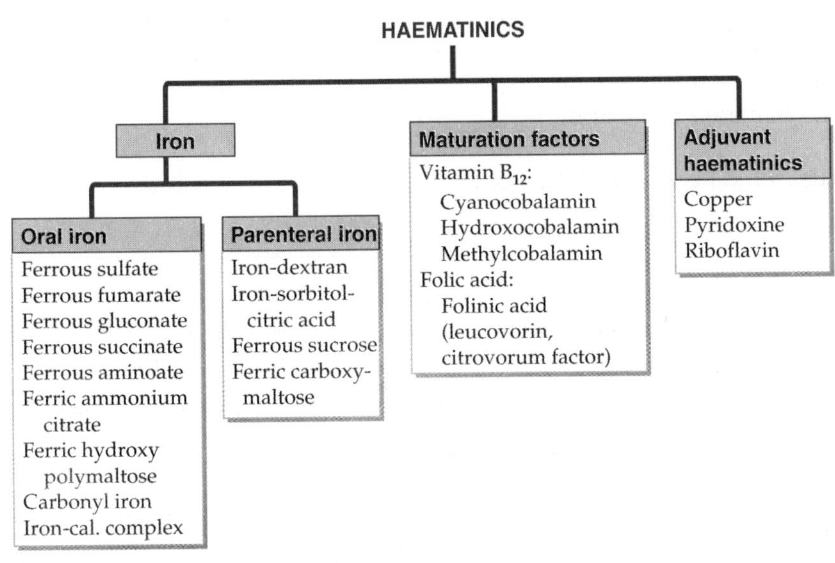

Preparations

Oral iron: Therapeutic dose: 100–200 mg elemental iron per day (children 3–5 mg/kg/day). Prophylactic dose: 30 mg elemental iron (children 1 mg/kg) per day.

1. **Ferrous sulfate (hydrated salt 20% iron, dried salt 32% iron);** FERSOLATE 200 mg tab.
2. **Ferrous fumarate (33% iron);** NORI-A 200 mg tab.
3. **Ferrous gluconate (12% iron);** FERRONICUM 300 mg tab, 400 mg/15 ml elixir.
4. **Colloidal ferric hydroxide (50% iron);** FERRI DROPS 50 mg/ml oral drops.

Combination oral iron preparations

Trade name	*Iron compound*	*Other ingredients*
CONVIRON Cap	Fe. sulfate (dried) 60 mg	B_{12} 15 µg, folic acid 1.5 mg, B_6 1.5 mg, vit. C 75 mg
FERSOLATE-CM Tab	Fe. sulfate (dried) 195 mg	Cu sulfate 2.6 mg, Mn sulfate 2 mg
FESOVIT-SPANSULE Cap	Fe. sulfate (dried) 150 mg	B_{12} 15 µg, folic acid 1 mg, nicotinamide 50 mg, B_6 2 mg
FEFOL SPANSULE Cap	Fe. sulfate 150 mg	Folic acid 0.5 mg
HEMGLOB syr (15 ml)	Fe. gluconate 300 mg	B_{12} 15 µg, B_1 5 mg, B_2 5 mg, B_6 1.5 mg, niacinamide 45 mg
AUTRIN Cap	Fe. fumarate 300 mg	B_{12} 15 µg, folic acid 1.5 mg, vit. C 150 mg
DUMASULES Cap	Fe. fumarate 300 mg	B_{12} 7.5 µg, folic acid 0.75 mg, B_1 5 mg, niacinamide 50 mg, vit. C 75 mg, B_6 1.5 mg

Contd...

Contd...

HEMSYNERAL Cap	Fe. fumarate 200 mg	B_{12} 15 µg, folic acid 1.5 mg
HEMSI Syr (5 ml)	Fe. fumarate 100 mg	Vit. B_{12} 5 µg, folic acid 0.5 mg, Zn 3.3 mg, Cu 0.035 mg, Mn 0.2 mg
HEMATRINE Cap	Fe. succinate 100 mg	B_{12} 2.5 µg, folic acid 0.5 mg, vit. C 25 mg, niacinamide 15 mg
POLYRON tab, BIOFER tab, POLYFER chewable tab	Iron hydroxy polymaltose (Iron 100 mg)	Folic acid 0.35 mg
MUMFER Syr (5 ml) and drops (1 ml)	Iron hydroxy polymaltose (Iron 50 mg)	Folic acid 0.5 mg
FERRICARB Cap	Carbonyl iron (Iron 100 mg)	Folic acid 1.5 mg, B_{12} 15 µg, Zinc sulf 88 mg, pyridoxin 3 mg, Sod. selenite 60 µg
HBFAST Tab	Carbonyl iron (Iron 100 mg)	Folic acid 0.35 mg
FERROCHELATE Syr (5 ml) drops (1 ml)	Ferric ammon. cit. (Iron 60 mg) (Iron 20 mg)	B_{12} 5 µg, folic acid 1 mg, B_{12} 4 µg, folic acid 0.2 mg
RARICAP Tab	Iron cal. complex (Iron 25 mg)	Folic acid 0.3 mg
PROBOFEX Cap	Fe. aminoate (60 mg Iron)	B_{12} 15 µg, folic acid 1.5 mg, B_6 3 mg
DEXORANGE Cap/ syrup (15 ml)	Ferric ammon. cit. 160 mg	B_{12} 7.5 µg, folic acid 0.5 mg.

Parenteral Iron

1. **Iron-dextran:** 50 mg elemental iron/ml in colloidal solution; 2 ml deep i.m. injection by 'Z' track technique, daily or on alternate days; 2 ml by slow i.v. injection (taking 10 min) daily;
   IMFERON, FERRI INJ: 2 ml amp.
2. **Iron-sorbitol-citric acid:** 50 mg elemental iron/ml; 1.5 ml daily or on alternate days by deep i.m. injection using 'Z' track technique;
   FERIMAX: iron sorbitol-citric acid 75 mg, folic acid 0.75 mg, hydroxocobalamine 75 µg in 1.5 ml Amp.
3. **Ferrous-sucrose:** 100 mg slow i.v. inj. over 5 min daily or on alternate days. Not for i.m. or s.c. inj;
   MICROFER, UNIFERON, ICOR 50 mg/2.5 ml and 100 mg/5 ml inj.
4. **Ferric-carboxymaltose:** 100 mg slow i.v. inj. daily or upto 1000 mg diluted in 100 ml saline and infused i.v. taking 15-30 min; infusion can be repeated after 1 week.
   ENCICARB INJ 50 mg/ml in 2 ml and 10 ml vials.

Maturation factors

1. **Cyanocobalamin/Hydroxocobalamin:** Therapeutic dose: 30–1000 µg/day by i.m. or deep s.c. injection (not i.v.) for 10 days followed by weekly and then monthly doses; Prophylactic dose 3–10 µg/day oral; available only as combined formulations with other vitamins and iron:

   NEUROBION FORTE (1000 µg/3 ml inj; 15 µg per tab), OPTINEURON (1000 µg/3 ml inj), NEUROXIN-12 (500 µg/10 ml inj), POLYBION (15 µg per cap), BECOSULES (5 µg/cap), AUTRIN (15 µg/cap).
2. **Methylcobalamin:** 0.5–1.5 mg/day oral;
   BIOCOBAL, DIACOBAL, METHYLCOBAL 0.5 mg tab, MECOBA, BIGVIN 500 µg/ml inj.
3. **Folic acid:** Therapeutic dose 2–5 mg/day oral/i.m.; prophylactic dose 0.5 mg/day;
   FOLVITE, FOLITAB 5 mg tab.

4. **Folinic acid:** 1–3 mg i.v.; CALCIUM LEUCOVORIN 3 mg/ml inj; FASTOVORIN 3 mg and 15 mg amps, 50 mg vial; RECOVORIN 15 mg tab, 15 mg and 30 mg vial for inj.

Erythropoietic factor

Recombinant human erythropoietin (Epoetin α, β): 25–100 IU/kg s.c./i.v. 3 times a week (max 600 IU/kg/week);
HEMAX 2000 IU/ml and 4000 IU/ml vials; EPREX 2000 IU, 4000 IU and 10,000 IU in 1 ml prefilled syringes; ZYROP (epoetin β) 2000 IU and 4000 IU vials.

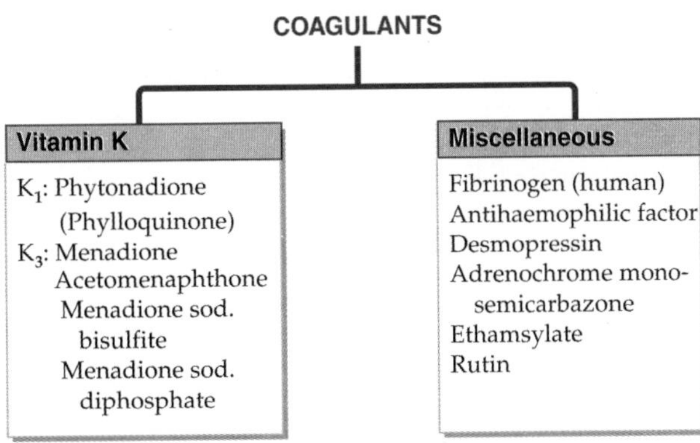

Preparations

1. **Vitamin K:** 5–10 mg oral/i.m. repeated as required;

   Phytonadione: VITAMIN-K, KVI, K-WIN 10 mg/ml for i.m. injection.

   Menadione: 0.66 mg in GYNAE CVP with vit C 75 mg, ferrous gluconate 67 mg, cal. lactate 300 mg and citras bioflavonoid 150 mg per cap.

   Acetomenaphthone: ACETOMENADIONE 5, 10 mg tab; KAPILIN 10 mg tab.

   Menadione sod. bisulfite: 20 mg, in CADISPER-C with vit C 100 mg, adrenochrome monosemicarbazone, 1 mg, rutin 60 mg, methylhesperidin 40 mg, cal. phosphate 100 mg per tab.
   STYPTOCID 10 mg with adrenochrome monosemicarbazone 0.5 mg, rutin 50 mg, vit C 37.5 mg, vit D 200 i.u., cal. phosphate 260 mg per tab.
2. **Fibrinogen:** 0.5 g by i.v. infusion; FIBRINAL 0.5 g Vac.
3. **Antihaemophilic factor:** 5–10 U/kg by i.v. infusion, repeated 6–12 hourly. FIBRINAL-H, ANTIHAEMOPHILIC FACTOR: 150 U or 200 U + fibrinogen 0.5 g/bottle for i.v. infusion.
4. **Adrenochrome monosemicarbazone:** 1–5 mg oral/i.m.; STYPTOCHROME 3 mg/2 ml inj.
5. **Rutin:** 60–200 mg BD–TDS oral/i.m.; In CADISPER-C 60 mg tab.
6. **Ethamsylate:** 250–500 mg TDS oral/i.v.;
   ETHAMSYL, DICYNENE, HEMSYL, K. STAT 250, 500 mg tabs; 250 mg/2 ml inj.

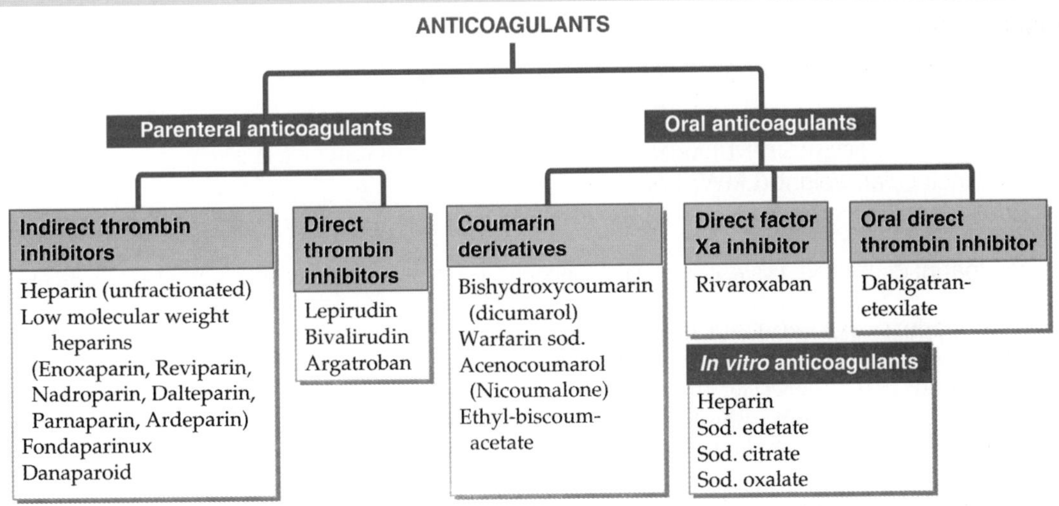
ANTICOAGULANTS
Parenteral anticoagulants
Oral anticoagulants
Indirect thrombin inhibitors
Heparin (unfractionated)
Low molecular weight heparins
(Enoxaparin, Reviparin, Nadroparin, Dalteparin, Parnaparin, Ardeparin)
Fondaparinux
Danaparoid
Direct thrombin inhibitors
Lepirudin
Bivalirudin
Argatroban
Coumarin derivatives
Bishydroxycoumarin (dicumarol)
Warfarin sod.
Acenocoumarol (Nicoumalone)
Ethyl-biscoum-acetate
Direct factor Xa inhibitor
Rivaroxaban
Oral direct thrombin inhibitor
Dabigatran-etexilate
In vitro anticoagulants
Heparin
Sod. edetate
Sod. citrate
Sod. oxalate

Preparations

1. **Heparin (unfractionated):** 5000–10,000 U (children 50–100 U/kg) i.v. bolus dose followed by 750–1000 U/hr i.v. infusion;

   Low dose (s.c.) regimen: 5000 U s.c. every 8–12 hours;
   HEPARIN SOD., BEPARINE, NUPARIN 1000 and 5000 U/ml in 5 ml vials for injection.

2. **Low molecular weight (LMW) heparins:**

   Enoxaparin: CLEXANE 20 mg (0.2 ml) and 40 mg (0.4 ml) prefilled syringes; 20–40 mg OD, s.c. (start 2 hour before surgery).

   Reviparin: CLIVARINE 13.8 mg (eq. to 1432 anti Xa IU) in 0.25 ml prefilled syringe; 0.25 ml s.c. once daily for 5–10 days.

   Nadroparin: FRAXIPARINE 3075 IU (0.3 ml) and 4100 IU (0.4 ml) inj., CARDIOPARIN 4000 anti Xa IU/0.4 ml, 6000 anti Xa IU/0.6 ml, 100,000 anti Xa IU/10 ml inj.

   Dalteparin: 2500 IU s.c. OD for prophylaxis; 100 U/Kg 12 hourly or 200 U/Kg 24 hourly s.c. for treatment of deep vein thrombosis. FRAGMIN 2500, 5000 IU prefilled syringes.

   Parnaparin: 0.6 ml s.c. OD for unstable angina and prophylaxis of DVT; FLUXUM 3200 IU (0.3 ml), 6400 IU (0.6 ml) inj.

   Ardeparin: 2500–5000 IU s.c. OD; INDEPARIN 2500 IU, 5000 IU prefilled syringes.

3. **Fondaparinux:** 5–10 mg s.c. once daily; FONDAPARINUX, ARIXTRA 5 mg/0.4 ml, 7.5 mg/0.6 ml and 10 mg/0.8 ml prefilled single dose syringe.

4. **Bishydroxycoumarin (Dicumarol):** 200 mg for 2 days followed by 50–100 mg/day oral; DICOUMAROL 50 mg tab.

5. **Warfarin sod. (racemic):** 5–10 mg followed by 2–10 mg/day;
   UNIWARFIN 1, 2, 5 mg tabs, WARF-5 5 mg tab.

6. **Acenocoumarol (Nicoumalone):** 8–12 mg followed by 2–8 mg/day; ACITROM, NISTROM 1, 2, 4 mg tabs.
7. **Ethylbiscoum acetate:** 900 mg followed by 300–600 mg/day.
8. **Sodium citrate:** 1.65 g for 350 ml of blood (for transfusion); ANTICOAGULANT ACID CITRATE DEXTROSE SOLUTION 2.2 g/100 ml (75 ml is used for 1 unit of blood).
9. **Sodium oxalate:** 10 mg for 1 ml blood (for blood counts etc.).
10. **Sodium edetate:** 2 mg for 1 ml blood (for investigations).

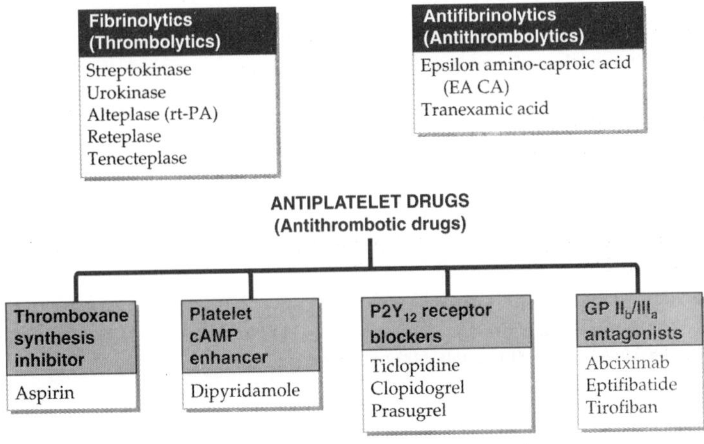

Fibrinolytics

1. **Streptokinase:** *For myocardial infarction:* 7.5–15 lac IU infused i.v. over 1 hr. *For deep vein thrombosis and pulmonary embolism:* 2.5 lac IU loading dose over 1/2–1 hr, followed by 1 lac IU/hr for 24 hr; STREPTASE, (freeze dried powder in vials) 2.5 lac, 7.5 lac and 15 lac IU/vial, ESKINASE, CARDIOSTREP 7.5 lac, 15 lac IU/vial.
2. **Urokinase:** *For myocardial infarction:* 2.5 lac IU i.v. over 10 min followed by 5 lac IU over next 60 min (stop in between if full recanalization occurs) or 6000 IU/min for upto 2 hr.

   For venous thrombosis and pulmonary embolism: 4400 IU/kg over 10 min i.v. followed by 4400 IU/kg/hr for 12 hr; UROKINASE, UROPASE, 2.5 lac, 5 lac, 7.5 lac, 10 lac IU per vial inj.
3. **Alteplase (recombinant tissue plasminogen activator (rt-PA):** *For MI:* 15 mg i.v. bolus injection followed by 50 mg over 30 min, then 35 mg over the next 1 hr. *For pulmonary embolism:* 100 mg i.v. infused over 2 hr; ACTILYSE 50 mg vial with 50 ml solvent water.
4. **Reteplase:** 10 mg i.v. over 10 min, repeat after 30 min.
5. **Tenecteplase:** 0.5 mg/kg single i.v. bolus injection. ELAXIM 30 mg, 50 mg per vial inj.

Antifibrinolytics

1. **Epsilon amino-caproic acid (EACA):** Initial priming dose is 5 g oral/i.v., followed by 1 g hourly till bleeding stops (max. 30 g in 24 hrs).

   AMICAR, HEMOCID, HAMOSTAT 0.5 g tab., 1.25 g/5 ml syr., 5 g/20 ml inj.
2. **Tranexamic acid:** 10–15 mg/kg 2–3 times a day or 1–1.5 g TDS oral, 0.5–1 g TDS by slow i.v. infusion. DUBATRAN, PAUSE, TRANAREST 500 mg tab, 500 mg/5 ml inj.

Antiplatelet Drugs

1. **Aspirin:** 75–150 mg OD oral; ASA 50 mg tab., COLSPRIN, DISPRIN CV–100: 100 mg soluble tab, LOPRIN 75 mg tab, ASPICOT 80 mg tab, ECOSPRIN 75, 150 mg tab.
2. **Dipyridamole:** 150–300 mg/day; PERSANTIN, 25, 100 mg tabs, THROMBONIL 75, 100 mg tabs; DYNASPRIN: dipyridamole 75 mg + aspirin 60 mg e.c. tab. CARDIWELL PLUS: dipyridamole 75 mg + aspirin 40 mg tab.
3. **Ticlopidine:** 250 mg BD with meals; TYKLID, TICLOVAS, TICLOP, 250 mg tab; ASTIC ticlopidine 250 mg + aspirin 100 mg tab.
4. **Clopidogrel:** 75 mg OD, CLODREL, CLOPILET, DEPLATT 75 mg tab; Clopidogrel 75 mg + aspirin 75 mg: CLODREL PLUS, CLOPITAB-A, THROMBOSPRIN, SYNPLATT tab.
5. **Prasugrel:** 10 mg OD: elderly and those below 60 kg body weight 5 mg OD; for urgent action 60 mg single loading dose; PRASULET, PRASUSAFE, PRASUREL 5 mg, 10 mg tabs.
6. **Abciximab:** (Glycoprotein II_b/III_a receptor antagonist) 0.25 mg/kg i.v. 10–60 min before PTCA, followed by 10 μg/min for 12 hr; REOPRO 2 mg/ml inj.
7. **Eptifibatide:** Initially 180 μg/kg/i.v. followed by 2 μg/kg/min i.v. infusion for upto 72 hours; CLOTIDE, UNIGRILIN, COROMAX 20 mg/10 ml and 75 mg/100 ml inj.
8. **Tirofiban:** Initially 0.4 μg/kg/min i.v. infusion for 30 min, followed by 0.1 μg/kg/min infusion for 48–108 hours. AGGRAMED, AGGRITOR, AGGRIBLOC 5 mg/100 ml infusion.

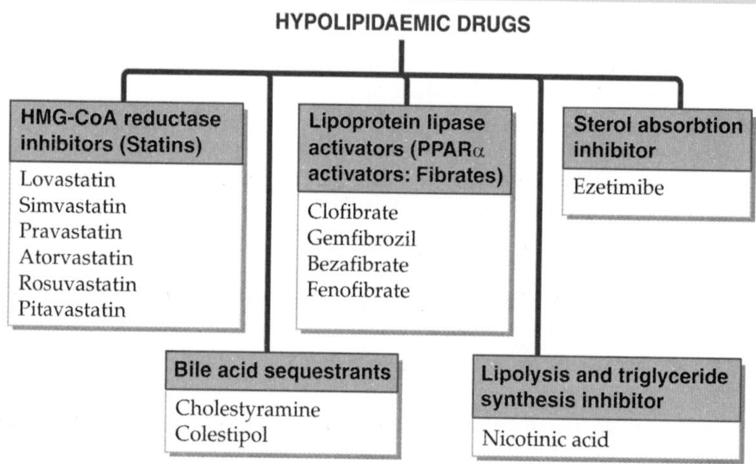

Preparations

1. **Lovastatin:** 10–40 mg/day; ROVACOR, AZTATIN, LOVAMEG 10, 20 mg tabs.
2. **Simvastatin:** 5–20 mg/day (max 80 mg); SIMVOTIN, SIMCARD, ZOSTA 5, 10, 20 mg tabs.
3. **Pravastatin:** 10–40 mg/day; PRAVATOR 10, 20 mg tabs.
4. **Atorvastatin:** 10–40 mg/day (max 80 mg); AZTOR, ATORVA, ATORLIP 5, 10, 20 mg tabs.
5. **Rosuvastatin:** 5–20 mg/day (max. 40 mg/day); ROSUVAS, ROSYN 5, 10, 20 mg tab.

6. **Pitavastatin:** 1–4 mg/day; FLOVAS 1.0, 2.0 mg tabs.
7. **Gemfibrozil:** 600 mg BD; GEMPAR, NORMOLIP, 300 mg cap., LOPID 300 mg cap, 600 mg and 900 mg tabs.
8. **Bezafibrate:** 200 mg TDS with meals; BEZALIP 200 mg tab, 400 mg (retard) tab.
9. **Fenofibrate:** 200 mg OD with meals; FENOLIP, LIPICARD 200 mg cap.
10. **Nicotinic acid:** Start with 100 mg TDS, gradually increase to 2–6 g per day in divided doses. It should be taken just after food to minimize flushing and itching;
    NIALIP, NEASYN-SR, 375, 500 mg tabs.
11. **Ezetimibe:** 10 mg OD; ZETICA, EZEDOC 10 mg tab.

    Ezetimibe 10 mg + atorvastatin 10 mg: BITORVA, LIPIVAS-EZ, LIPONORM-EZ;
    Ezetimibe 10 mg + simvastatin 10 mg: STARSTAT-EZ, SIMVAS-EZ.

Plasma Expanders

1. **Human Albumin:** 5–20% by i.v. infusion; ALBUDAC, ALBUPAN (20%) 50, 100 ml inj., ALBUMED 5%, 20% infusion (100 ml).
2. **Dextran-70 (MW 70,000):** 6% by i.v. infusion; DEXTRAN-70, LOMODEX- 70; 6% solution in dextrose or saline, 540 ml vac.

   Dextran-40 (MW 40,000; low MW dextran): 10% by i.v. infusion LOMODEX 10% solution in dextrose or saline, 540 ml vac.
3. **Polygeline (degraded gelatin polymer):** 3.5% by i.v. infusion; HAEMACCEL, SERACCEL 500 ml vac. (as 3.5% solution in balanced electrolyte medium).
4. **Hetastarch:** 6% by i.v. infusion; EXPAN 6% in 100, 500 ml vac.

10 Gastrointestinal Drugs

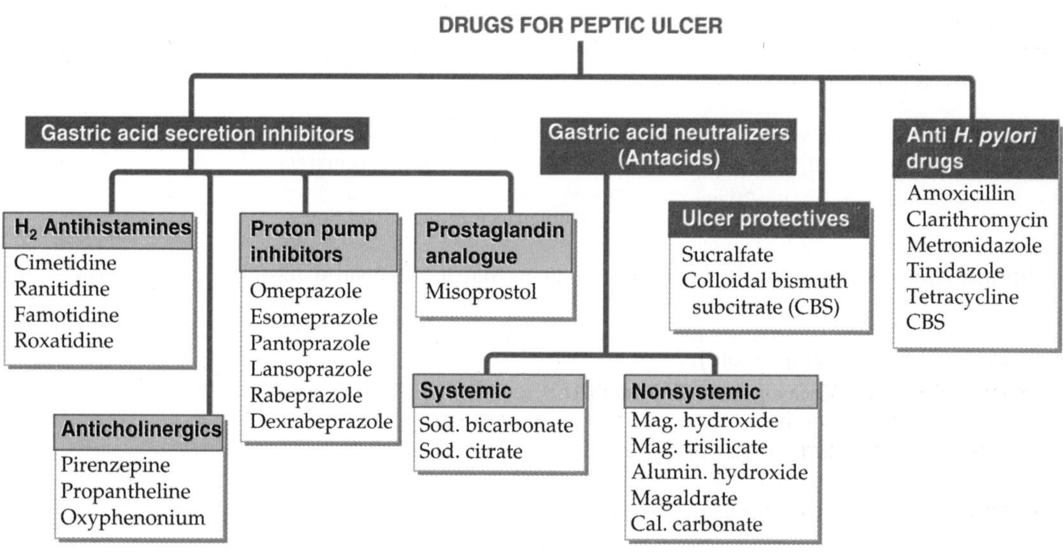

Preparations

1. **Cimetidine:** 400 mg BD or 800 mg OD at bed time, 50 mg/hour i.v. infusion; CIMETIDINE, 200 mg, 400 mg, 800 mg tabs, 200 mg/2 ml inj.
2. **Ranitidine:** *For ulcer healing*–150 mg BD or 300 mg at bed time; *For prevention of ulcer recurrence*–150 mg at bed time; *For Zollinger-Ellison syndrome*–300 mg TDS or QID; Parenteral dose 50 mg i.m. or slow i.v. injection every 6–8 hours or 0.1–0.25 mg/kg/hr i.v. infusion; ULTAC, ZINETAC 150 mg, 300 mg tabs; HISTAC, RANTAC, RANITIN, ACILOC 150 mg, 300 mg tabs, 50 mg/2 ml inj.
3. **Famotidine:** 40 mg at bed time or 20 mg BD (for healing); 20 mg at bed time for maintenance; upto 480 mg/day in ZE syndrome; parenteral dose 20 mg i.v. 12 hourly, or 2 mg/hr i.v. infusion. FAMTAC, FAMONITE, TOPCID 20 mg, 40 mg tabs; FAMOCID, FACID 20, 40 mg tabs, 20 mg/2 ml inj.
4. **Roxatidine:** 150 mg at bed time or 75 mg BD; maintenance 75 mg at bed time. ROTANE, ZORPEX 75 mg, 150 mg SR tabs.
5. **Omeprazole:** 20–60 mg/day, ZE syndrome 60–120 mg/day in two divided doses; OMIZAC, NILSEC 20 mg cap. OMEZ, OCID, OMEZOL 10, 20 mg caps, PROTOLOC 20, 40 mg caps containing enteric coated granules. Capsules must not be opened or chewed; to be taken in the morning before meals.

   Esomeprazole (s-omeprazole): 20–40 mg OD; NEXPRO, RACIPER, IZRA 20, 40 mg tab.
6. **Lansoprazole:** Ulcer healing dose: 15–30 mg OD; LANZOL, LANZAP, LEVANT, LANPRO 15, 30 mg caps.
7. **Pantoprazole:** 40 mg OD; PANTOCID, PANTODAC 20, 40 mg enteric coated tab; PANTIUM, PANTIN 40 mg tab, 40 mg inj for i.v. use.

   S(-) Pantoprazole: 20 mg OD; PANPURE, ZOSECTA 20 mg tab.
8. **Rabeprazole:** 20 mg OD, ZE syndrome 60 mg/day; RABLET, RAZO, RABLOC, RABICIP, HAPPI 10, 20 mg tab, 20 mg/ml vial for inj.

9. **Dexrabeprazole:** 10–20 mg OD; DEXPURE, 5, 10 mg tabs.
10. **Misoprostol (Methyl PGE_1 ester):** 200 μg QID; CYTOLOG 200 μg tab; MISOPROST 100 μg, 200 μg tabs.
11. **Magnesium hydroxide:** 0.4–1.0 g as often as required; MILK OF MAGNESIA 0.4 g/5 ml suspension.
12. **Aluminium hydroxide gel:** 0.6–2.4 g as required; ALUDROX 0.84 g tab, 0.6 g/10 ml suspension.
13. **Magaldrate:** 0.4–0.8 g as required; STACID 400 mg tab, 400 mg/5 ml susp; ULGEL 400 mg with 20 mg simethicone per tab or 5 ml susp.
14. **Combination antacid preparations**

ACIDIN: Mag. carb. 165 mg, dried alum. hydrox. gel 232 mg, cal. carb. 165 mg, sod. bicarb. 82 mg, with kaolin 105 mg and belladonna herb 30 μg per tab.

ALMACARB: Dried alum. hydrox. gel 325 mg, mag. carb. 50 mg, methyl polysilox. 40 mg, deglycyrrhizinated liquorice 380 mg per tab.

ALLUJEL-DF: Dried alum. hydrox. gel 400 mg, mag. hydrox. 400 mg, methyl polysilox. 30 mg per 10 ml susp.

DIGENE: Dried alum. hydrox. gel 300 mg, mag. alum. silicate 50 mg, mag. hydrox. 25 mg, methylpolysilox. 10 mg per tab.

DIGENE GEL: Mag. hydrox. 185 mg, alum. hydrox. gel 830 mg, sod. carboxymethyl cellulose 100 mg, methylpolysilox. 25 mg per 10 ml susp.

GELUSIL: Dried alum. hydrox. gel 250 mg, mag. trisilicate 500 mg per tab.

GELUSIL LIQUID: Mag. trisilicate 625 mg, alum. hydrox. gel 312 mg per 5 ml susp.

MUCAINE: Alum. hydrox. 290 mg, mag. hydrox. 98 mg, oxethazaine 10 mg per 5 ml susp.

TRICAINE-MPS: Alum. hydrox. gel 300 mg, mag. hydrox. 150 mg, oxethazaine 10 mg, simethicone 10 mg per 5 ml gel.

MAYLOX: Dried alum. hydrox. gel 225 mg, mag. hydrox. 200 mg, dimethicone 50 mg per tab and 5 ml susp.

POLYCROL FORTE GEL: Mag. hydrox. 100 mg, dried alum. hydrox. gel 425 mg, methylpolysilox. 125 mg per 5 ml susp.

15. **Sucralfate:** Ulcer healing dose: 1 g taken 1 hour before 3 major meals and at bed time; To prevent recurrences 1 g BD; SUCRACE, ULCERFATE, RECULFATE 1 g tab.
16. **Colloidal bismuth subcitrate (CBS, Tripotassium dicitrato-bismuthate):** 120 mg (as Bi_2O_3) taken 30 min before 3 major meals and at bed time; TRYMO, DENOL 120 mg tab.

Anti-H. pylori antimicrobials

Amoxicillin:	750–1000 mg BD
Clarithromycin:	500 mg BD
Tetracycline:	500 mg QID
Metronidazole:	400 mg TDS
Tinidazole:	500 mg BD

Regimens consist of two of the above antimicrobials taken along with a proton pump inhibitor for 1–3 weeks.

Anti-*H. pylori* kits (one kit to be taken daily in 2 doses)

HP-KIT, HELIBACT, OMXITIN: Omeprazole 20 mg 2 cap + Amoxicillin 750 mg 2 tab + Tinidazole 500 mg 2 tab.
PYLOMOX: Lansoprazole 15 mg 2 cap + Amoxicillin 750 mg 2 tab + Tinidazole 500 mg 2 tab.
LANSI KIT: Lansoprazole 30 mg 1 cap + Amoxicillin 750 mg 1 tab + Tinidazole 500 mg 1 tab (one kit twice a day)
PYLOKIT, HELIGO: Lansoprazole 30 mg 2 cap + Clarithromycin 250 mg 2 cap + Tinidazole 500 mg 2 tab.
LANPRO AC: Lansoprazole 30 mg 2 cap + Clarithromycin 250 mg 2 tab + Amoxicillin 750 mg 2 tab.

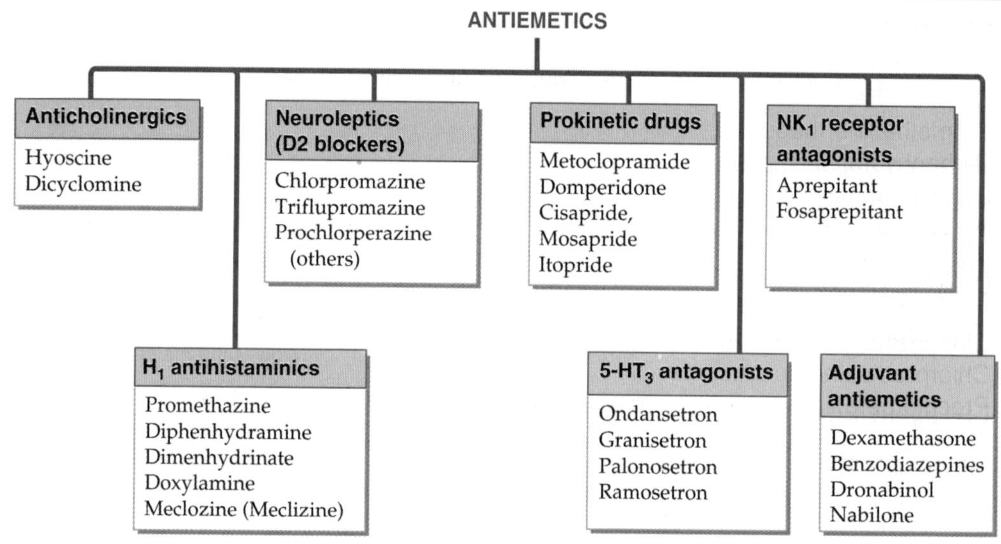
ANTIEMETICS
Anticholinergics
Hyoscine
Dicyclomine
Neuroleptics (D2 blockers)
Chlorpromazine
Triflupromazine
Prochlorperazine (others)
Prokinetic drugs
Metoclopramide
Domperidone
Cisapride,
Mosapride
Itopride
NK1 receptor antagonists
Aprepitant
Fosaprepitant
H1 antihistaminics
Promethazine
Diphenhydramine
Dimenhydrinate
Doxylamine
Meclozine (Meclizine)
5-HT3 antagonists
Ondansetron
Granisetron
Palonosetron
Ramosetron
Adjuvant antiemetics
Dexamethasone
Benzodiazepines
Dronabinol
Nabilone

Preparations

1. Hyoscine: 0.2–0.4 mg oral/i.m./transdermal patch.
2. Dicyclomine: 10–20 mg oral.
3. Promethazine theoclate: 25–50 mg oral; AVOMINE 25 mg tab.
4. Diphenhydramine: 25–50 mg oral.
5. Dimenhydrinate: 25–50 mg oral.
6. Meclozine: 25–50 mg oral; PREGNIDOXIN: Meclozine 25 mg + caffeine 20 mg tab; DILIGAN: Meclozine 12.5 mg + nicotinic acid 50 mg.
7. Doxylamine: 10–20 mg at bed time (for morning sickness); DOXINATE, GRAVIDOX, VOMNEX, NOSIC 10 mg tab (with pyridoxine 10 mg)
8. Cinnarizine: 25–50 mg oral.
9. Chlorpromazine: 10–25 mg oral/i.m.
10. Prochlorperazine: 5–10 mg BD/TDS oral, 12.5–25 mg by deep i.m. inj.; STEMETIL 5 mg tab, 12.5 mg/ml inj in 1 ml amp, VOMTIL 5 mg tab.
11. Metoclopramide: 10 mg (children 0.25–0.5 mg/kg) TDS oral or i.m. For chemotherapy induced vomiting 0.3–2.0 mg/kg i.v./i.m; PERINORM, MAXERON, REGLAN, SIGMET, 10 mg tab; 5 mg/5 ml syr; 10 mg/2 ml inj.; 50 mg/10 ml inj.
12. Domperidone: 10–40 mg (Children 0.3–0.6 mg/kg) TDS; DOMSTAL, DOMPERON, NORMETIC 10 mg tab, 1 mg/ml susp, MOTINORM 10 mg tab, 10 mg/ml drops.
13. Mosapride: 5 mg (elderly 2.5 mg) TDS; MOZA, MOZASEF, MOPRIDE 2.5 mg, 5 mg tabs; MOZA MPS: 5 mg + methylpolysiloxane 125 mg tab.
14. Itopride: 50 mg TDS; ITOFLUX, ITOKINE, ITOPRID, GANATON 50 mg tab.

15. **Ondansetron:** For cisplatin and other highly emetogenic drugs—8 mg i.v. by slow injection over 15 min ½ hr before chemotherapeutic infusion, followed by 2 similar doses 4 hour apart. To prevent delayed emesis 8 mg oral is given twice a day for 3–5 days. For postoperative nausea/vomiting 4–8 mg i.v. given before induction is repeated 8 hourly. For less emetogenic drugs and for radiotherapy an oral dose of 8 mg is given 1–2 hr prior to the procedure and repeated twice 8 hrly.
    EMESET, VOMIZ, OSETRON, EMSETRON 4, 8 mg tabs, 2 mg/ml inj in 2 ml and 4 ml amps; ONDY, EMESET 2 mg/5 ml syr.
16. **Granisetron:** 1–3 mg diluted in 20–50 ml saline and infused i.v. over 5 min before chemotherapy, repeated after 12 hr. For less emetogenic regimen 2 mg oral 1 hr before chemotherapy or 1 mg before and 1 mg 12 hr after it. For post-operative vomiting 1 mg diluted in 5 ml and slowly injected i.v. followed by 1 mg orally every 12 hours. GRANICIP, GRANISET 1 mg, 2 mg tabs; 1 mg/ml inj. (1 ml and 3 ml amps).
17. **Palonosetron:** 250 μg by slow i.v. inj 30 min before chemotherapy; not to be repeated before 7 days. For post-operative vomiting 75 μg single injection. PALONOX 0.25 mg/ml inj; PALZEN 0.25 mg/50 ml inj.
18. **Ramosetron:** 0.3 mg i.v. before chemotherapy or surgery, may be repeated once daily, 0.1 mg oral for less emetogenic chemotherapy; NOZIA 0.1 mg tab, 0.3 mg in 2 ml amp.
19. **Aprepitant:** 125 mg oral before chemotherapy and 80 mg on 2nd and 3rd day alongwith i.v. ondansetron + dexamethasone. For postoperative vomiting 40 mg single oral dose before surgery;
    APRECAP, APRESET, APRELIFE 125 mg (one cap) + 80 mg (2 caps) Kit.
20. **Dexamethasone:** 8–20 mg i.v. 1/2–1 hour before emetogenic chemotherapy, generally to supplement metoclopramide/ondansetron.
21. **Diazepam:** 5–10 mg oral to supplement metoclopramide/ondansetron.
22. **Dronabinol:** 5–10 mg/m^2 body surface area orally for moderately emetogenic chemotherapy in patients non-responsive to other drugs.

Note: *See* Index for preparations of other drugs.

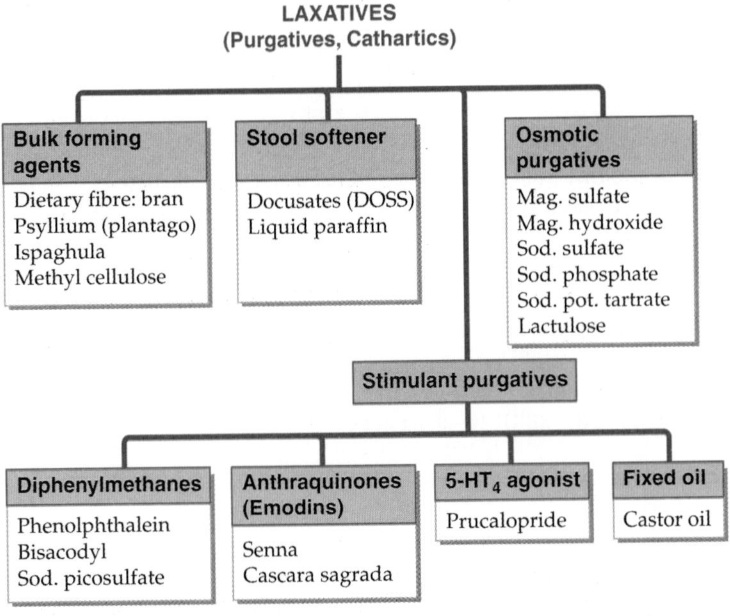
LAXATIVES
(Purgatives, Cathartics)
Bulk forming agents
Dietary fibre: bran
Psyllium (plantago)
Ispaghula
Methyl cellulose
Stool softener
Docusates (DOSS)
Liquid paraffin
Osmotic purgatives
Mag. sulfate
Mag. hydroxide
Sod. sulfate
Sod. phosphate
Sod. pot. tartrate
Lactulose
Stimulant purgatives
Diphenylmethanes
Phenolphthalein
Bisacodyl
Sod. picosulfate
Anthraquinones (Emodins)
Senna
Cascara sagrada
5-HT4 agonist
Prucalopride
Fixed oil
Castor oil

Preparations

1. **Psyllium hydrophilic mucilloid:** 6–12 g to be taken just after mixing with water; ISOVAC 65 g/100 g granules.
2. **Ispaghula (refined husk):** 3–12 g freshly mixed with water or milk 2–3 times a day; ISOGEL (27 g/30 g), NATURE CURE (49 g/100 g), FYBOGEL (3.5 g/5.4 g) powder FIBRIL (3.4 g/11 g) powder.
3. **Methyl cellulose:** 4–6 g/day mixed with water.
4. **Docusates (Dioctyl sodium sulfosuccinate, DOSS):** 100–400 mg/day; CELLUBRIL 100 mg cap; LAXICON 100 mg tab, DOSLAX 150 mg cap. As enema 50–150 mg in 50–100 ml; LAXICON 125 mg in 50 ml enema.
5. **Liquid paraffin:** 15–30 ml/day as such or in emulsified form.
6. **Phenolphthalein:** 60–130 mg; LAXIL 130 mg tab. To be taken at bedtime (tab. not to be chewed).
7. **Bisacodyl:** 5–15 mg; DULCOLAX 5 mg tab; 10 mg (adult) 5 mg (child) suppository; CONLAX 5 mg, 10 mg suppository, BIDLAX-5 5 mg tab.
8. **Sodium picosulfate:** 5-10 mg at bed time; CREMALAX, LAXICARE 10 mg tab, PICOFIT 5 mg/5 ml syr.
9. **Senna (as Sennosides Cal. salt):** 10–40 mg at bed time: GLAXENNA 11.5 mg tab; PURSENNID 18 mg tab; SOFSENA 12 mg tab.
10. **Mag. sulfate (Epsom salt):** 5–15 g dissolved in 150–200 ml water, taken in the morning.
11. **Mag. hydroxide** (as 8% W/W suspension—milk of magnesia) 30 ml.
12. **Sod. sulfate (Glauber's salt):** 10–15 g dissolved in 150–200 ml water, taken in the morning.
13. **Sod. phosphate:** 6–12 g dissolved in 150–200 ml water, taken in the morning.
14. **Sod. pot. tartrate (Rochelle salt):** 8–15 g dissolved in 150–200 ml water, taken in the morning.

15. **Lactulose:** 10 g BD taken with water;
LACSAN, MTLAC 10 g/ 15 ml liquid, DUPHALAC, LIVOLUK 6.67 g/10 ml liq.

Some combined preparations

AGAROL: Liquid paraffin 9.5 ml, phenolphthalein 400 mg, agar 60 mg per 30 ml emulsion.
CREMAFFIN: Milk of magnesia 11.25 ml, liq. paraffin 3.75 ml per 15 ml emulsion; CREMAFFIN PINK with phenolphthalein 50 mg per 15 ml.
JULAX: Bisacodyl 10 mg, casanthranol 10 mg dragees.
PURSENNID-IN (with DOS): Purified senna ext. (cal salt) 18 mg, docusates 50 mg tab.

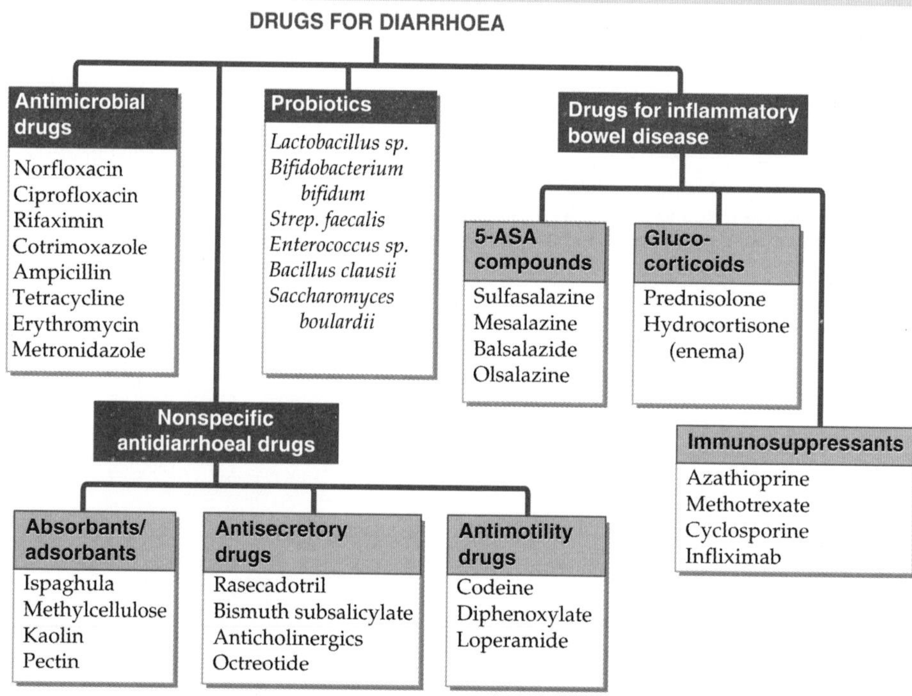
DRUGS FOR DIARRHOEA
Antimicrobial drugs
Norfloxacin
Ciprofloxacin
Rifaximin
Cotrimoxazole
Ampicillin
Tetracycline
Erythromycin
Metronidazole
Probiotics
Lactobacillus sp.
Bifidobacterium bifidum
Strep. faecalis
Enterococcus sp.
Bacillus clausii
Saccharomyces boulardii
Drugs for inflammatory bowel disease
5-ASA compounds
Sulfasalazine
Mesalazine
Balsalazide
Olsalazine
Gluco-corticoids
Prednisolone
Hydrocortisone (enema)
Immunosuppressants
Azathioprine
Methotrexate
Cyclosporine
Infliximab
Nonspecific antidiarrhoeal drugs
Absorbants/ adsorbants
Ispaghula
Methylcellulose
Kaolin
Pectin
Antisecretory drugs
Rasecadotril
Bismuth subsalicylate
Anticholinergics
Octreotide
Antimotility drugs
Codeine
Diphenoxylate
Loperamide

Preparations

1. **Rifaximin:** For traveller's diarrhoea 200 mg TDS for 3 days. For suppressing ammonia forming gut bacteria 550 mg TDS. RIFAGUT 200 mg, 550 mg tabs; TORFIX, RACFAX 200 mg tab.
2. **Probiotics:**
   - ECONORM, STIBS: *Saccharomyces boulardii* 250 mg sachet.
   - BIFILAC: *Lactobacillus* 50 million (M), *Streptococcus faecalis* 30M, *Clostridium butyricum* 2M, *Bacillus mesentericus* 1M per cap/sachet.
   - BIFILIN: *Lactobacillus sp.* 1 billion (B), *Bifidobacterium bifidum* 1B, *Streptococcus thermophillus* 0.25B, *Saccharomyces boulardii* 0.25B cap and sachet.
   - ACTIGUT: *Lactobacillus sp., Bifidobacterium sp.* cap.
   - ENTEROGERMINA: *Bacillus claussi* 2B spores/5 ml oral amp.
3. **Sulfasalazine (Salicylazosulfapyridine):** For inflammatory bowel disease—Remission inducing dose 3–4 g/day, maintenance dose 1.5–2 g/day oral; SALAZOPYRIN, SAZO-EN 0.5 g tab.
4. **Mesalazine (Mesalamine):** 1.2–2.4 g/day oral; 4 g by retention enema; MESACOL 0.4 g and 0.8 g tab, 0.5 g suppository; ASACOL, TIDOCOL 0.4 g tab, ETISA 0.5 g sachet; MESACOL ENEMA 4 g/60 ml.
5. **Balsalazide:** 1.5 g BD-2.25 g TDS; COLOREX 750 mg cap and per 5 ml syr., INTAZIDE 0.75 g tab.
6. **Racecadotril:** 100 mg (children 1.5 mg/kg) TDS for a maximum of 7 days; CADOTRIL, RACIGYL 100 mg cap, 15 mg sachet, REDOTIL 100 mg cap, ZEDOTT, ZOMATRIL 100 mg cap, 10 mg and 30 mg sachets and dispersible tabs.
7. **Codeine:** 60 mg TDS oral.
8. **Diphenoxylate-atropine:** LOMOTIL 2.5 mg diphenoxylate + 0.025 mg atropine per tab and 5 ml liquid; 2–4 tab followed by 1–2 tab 6 hourly.
9. **Loperamide:** 4 mg followed by 2 mg after each motion (max. 10 mg in a day); 2 mg BD for chronic diarrhoea. IMODIUM, LOPESTAL, DIARLOP: 2 mg tab, cap.

Note: *See* Index for preparations of other drugs

11 Antibacterial Drugs

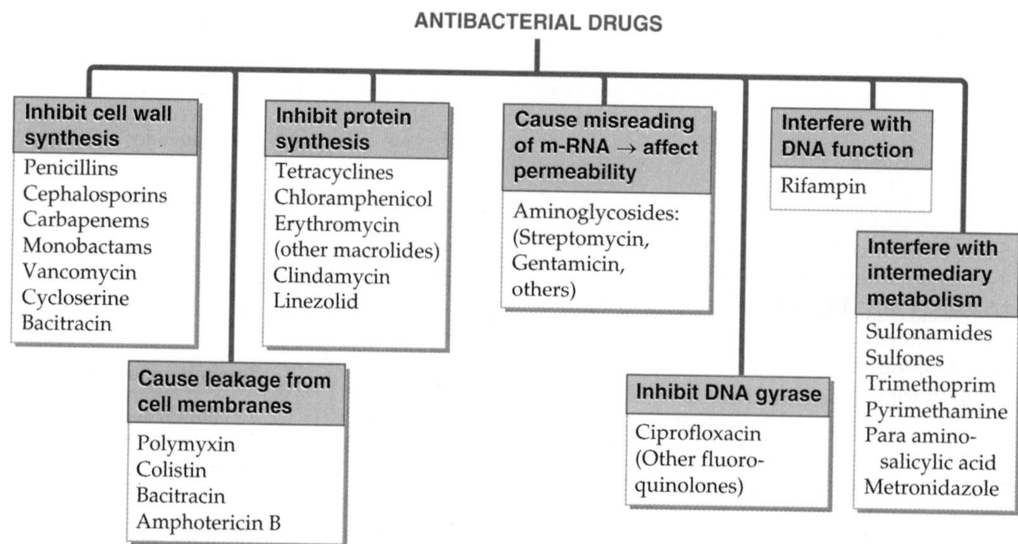

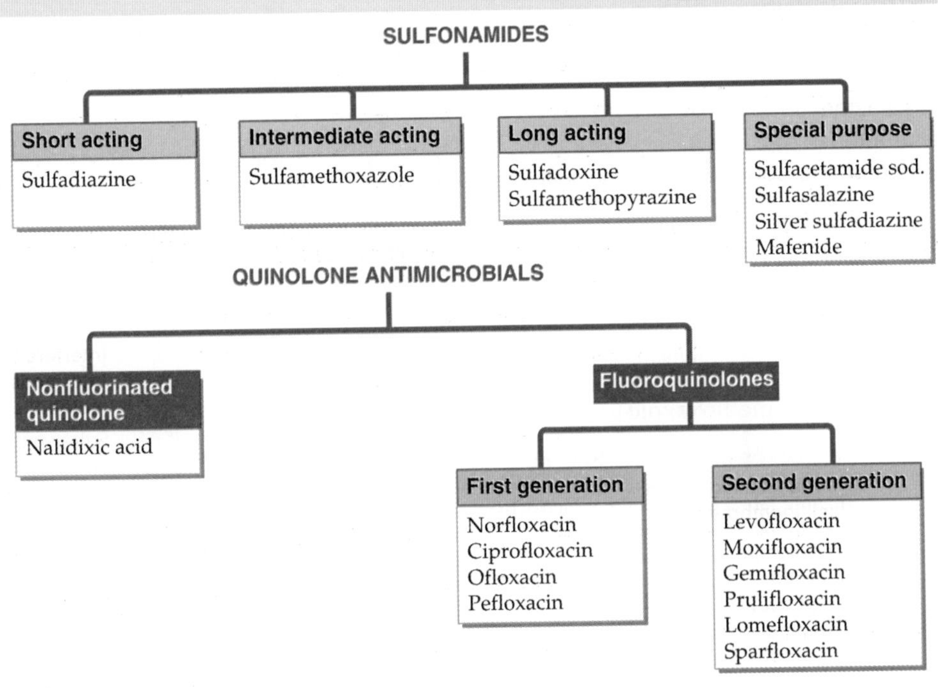
SULFONAMIDES
Short acting
Sulfadiazine
Intermediate acting
Sulfamethoxazole
Long acting
Sulfadoxine
Sulfamethopyrazine
Special purpose
Sulfacetamide sod.
Sulfasalazine
Silver sulfadiazine
Mafenide
QUINOLONE ANTIMICROBIALS
Nonfluorinated quinolone
Nalidixic acid
Fluoroquinolones
First generation
Norfloxacin
Ciprofloxacin
Ofloxacin
Pefloxacin
Second generation
Levofloxacin
Moxifloxacin
Gemifloxacin
Prulifloxacin
Lomefloxacin
Sparfloxacin

Preparations

Sulfonamides

1. **Sulfadiazine:** 0.5–2.0 g TDS; SULFADIAZINE 0.5 g tab.
2. **Sulfamethoxazole:** 1 g BD for 2 days, then 0.5 g BD; GANTANOL 0.5 g tab.
3. **Sulfacetamide sodium:** 6%–30% topically in the eye;
   LOCULA, ALBUCID 10%, 20%, 30% eye drops, 6% eye oint.
4. **Mafenide:** 1% topical application; SULFAMYLON 1% skin cream.
5. **Silver sulfadiazine:** 1% topical application;
   SILVIRIN 1% cream, ARGENEX 1% cream with chlorhexidine 0.2%.

Note: *See* Index for preparations of other sulfonamides.

Cotrimoxazole

(Trimethoprim-Sulfamethoxazole 1:5)

SEPTRAN, SEPMAX, BACTRIM, CIPLIN, ORIPRIM, SUPRISTOL, FORTRIM

Trimethoprim	*Sulfamethoxazole*
80 mg +	400 mg tab: 2 BD for 2 days then 1 BD.
160 mg +	800 mg tab: double strength (DS); 1 BD.
20 mg +	100 mg pediatric tab.
40 mg +	200 mg per 5 ml susp; infant 2.5 ml (not to be used in new borns), children 1–5 yr 5 ml, 6–12 year 10 ml (all BD).
160 mg +	800 mg per 3 ml for i.m. injection 12 hourly. (CIPLIN, ORIPRIM-IM)
80 mg +	400 mg per 5 ml for i.v. injection (WK-TRIM, ORIPRIM-IV) 10–15 ml BD.

Cotrimazine (Trimethoprim-Sulfadiazine 1:5)

Trimethoprim	*Sulfadiazine*
90 mg +	410 mg:AUBRIL tab and per 10 ml susp.; 2 tab BD for 2 days, then 1 BD.
180 mg +	820 mg: TRIGLOBE FORTE tabs.

Quinolones Antimicrobials

1. Nalidixic acid: 0.5–1 g TDS or QID oral; GRAMONEG 0.5 g tab, 0.3 g/5 ml susp, DIARLOP 0.3 g/5 ml susp.
2. Ciprofloxacin: 250–750 mg BD oral, 100–200 mg i.v. by slow infusion; 0.3% topically in eye; CIFRAN, CIPLOX, CIPROBID, QUINTOR, CIPROLET 250, 500, 750 mg tab, 200 mg/100 ml i.v. infusion, 3 mg/ml eye drops.
3. Ofloxacin: 200–400 mg BD oral, 200 mg by slow i.v. infusion; 0.3% topically in eye ZANOCIN, TARIVID, OFLOX 100, 200, 400 mg tab; 200 mg/100 ml i.v. infusion, ZENFLOX also 50 mg/5 ml susp., EXOCIN, OFLOX 0.3% eye drops.
4. Norfloxacin: 200–400 mg BD oral, 0.3% topically in eye; NORBACTIN, NORFLOX 200, 400, 800 mg tab, 100 mg/5 ml susp., 3 mg/ml eye drops. UROFLOX, NORILET 200, 400 mg tab, BACIGYL 400 mg tab, 400 mg/5 ml susp.
5. Pefloxacin: 400 mg BD oral, 400 mg i.v. by slow infusion; PELOX 200, 400 mg tab, to be taken with meals; 400 mg/5 ml inj (to be diluted in 100–250 ml of glucose solution but not saline), PERTI 400 mg tab.
6. Levofloxacin: 500 mg OD oral, 500 mg by slow i.v. infusion; TAVANIC, LEVOFLOX, LEVODAY, GLEVO 250, 500 mg tab, 500 mg/100 ml inj.
7. Lomefloxacin: 400 mg OD oral; LOMEF-400, LOMEDON, LOMADAY, LOMIBACT, LOX 400 mg tab, 0.3% eye drops.
8. Sparfloxacin: 200–400 mg OD oral; TOROSPAR 200, 400 mg tab, SPARTA, SPARQUIN, SPARDAC 100, 200 mg tab, ZOSPAR, EYPAR 0.3% eye drops.
9. Moxifloxacin: 400 mg OD oral; MOXIF 400 mg tab, STAXOM 400 mg tab, 400 mg/250 ml i.v. infusion, VIGAMOX, MOXICIP 0.5% eye drops.
10. Gemifloxacin: 320 mg OD for 5-7 days; TOPGEM, ZEMI, GEMBAX, GEMETOP 320 mg tab.
11. Prulifloxacin: 600 mg OD; ALPRULI, PRULIFLOX, PRULIFACT 600 mg tab.

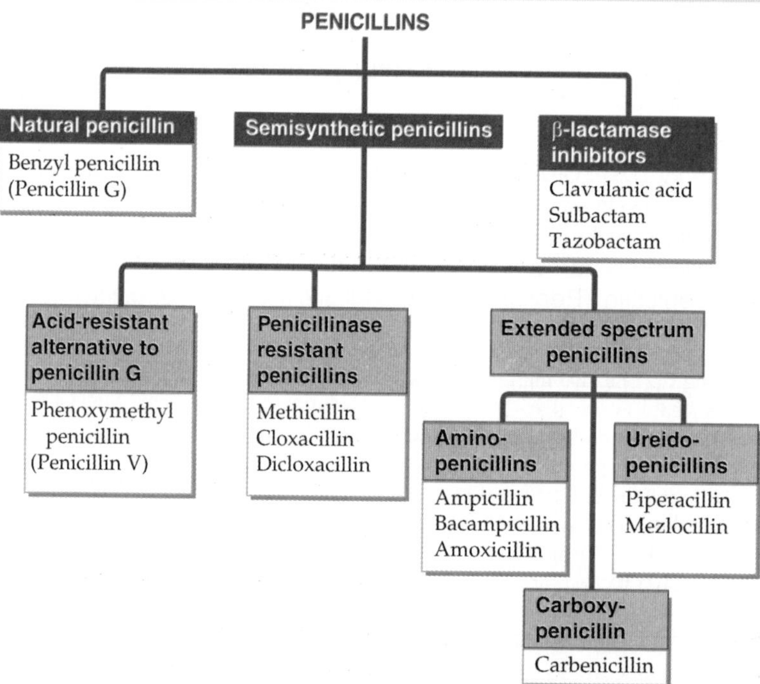
PENICILLINS
Natural penicillin
Benzyl penicillin (Penicillin G)
Semisynthetic penicillins
β-lactamase inhibitors
Clavulanic acid
Sulbactam
Tazobactam
Acid-resistant alternative to penicillin G
Phenoxymethyl penicillin (Penicillin V)
Penicillinase resistant penicillins
Methicillin
Cloxacillin
Dicloxacillin
Extended spectrum penicillins
Amino-penicillins
Ampicillin
Bacampicillin
Amoxicillin
Ureido-penicillins
Piperacillin
Mezlocillin
Carboxy-penicillin
Carbenicillin

Preparations

1. **Sod. penicillin G (crystalline penicillin) injection:** 0.5–5 MU i.m./i.v. 6–12 hourly. BENZYL PENICILLIN 0.5, 1.0 MU dry powder in vial to be dissolved in sterile water at the time of injection.
2. **Procaine penicillin G inj:** 0.5–1 MU i.m. 12–24 hourly as aqueous suspension; PROCAINE PENICILLIN-G 0.5, 1 MU dry powder in vial.
3. **Fortified procaine penicillin G inj:** contains 3 lac U procaine penicillin and 1 lac U sod. penicillin G, FORTIFIED P.P. INJ 3+1 lac U vial.
4. **Benzathine penicillin G:** 0.6–2.4 MU i.m. every 2–4 weeks as aqueous suspension. PENIDURE-LA (long acting), LONGACILLIN, PENCOM, 0.6, 1.2, 2.4 MU as dry powder in vial.
5. **Phenoxymethyl penicillin (Penicillin V):** 250–500 mg, infants 60 mg, children 125–250 mg; given 6 hourly, (250 mg = 4 lac U); CRYSTAPEN–V, KAYPEN, 125, 250 mg tab, 125 mg/5 ml dry syr—for reconstitution; PENIVORAL 65, 130 mg tab.
6. **Cloxacillin:** 0.25–0.5 g orally every 6 hours; for severe infections 0.25–1 g may be injected i.m. or i.v.—higher blood levels are produced; KLOX, BIOCLOX, 0.25, 0.5 g cap; 0.25, 0.5 g/vial inj. CLOPEN 0.25, 0.5 g cap.
7. **Ampicillin:** 0.5–2 g oral/i.m./i.v. depending on severity of infection, every 6 hours; children 50–100 mg/kg/day; AMPILIN, ROSCILLIN, BIOCILIN 250, 500 mg cap; 125, 250 mg/5 ml dry syr; 100 mg/ml pediatric drops; 250, 500 mg and 1.0 g per vial inj.
8. **Ampicillin + cloxacillin:** AMPILOX, DUOCLOX 250 + 250 mg cap, 500+500 mg DS tab, 125+125 mg kid tab and per 5 ml dry syr, 100 mg + 50 mg/ml pediatric syr, 250 mg + 250 mg per vial inj, 500 mg + 500 mg/vial DS inj, 125 mg + 125 mg/vial pediatric inj., 50 mg + 75 mg/vial neonatal inj.

9. **Bacampicillin:** 400–800 mg BD oral; PENGLOBE 200, 400 mg tabs.
10. **Amoxicillin:** 0.25–1 g TDS oral/i.m or slow i.v. injection, children 25–50 mg/kg/day; AMOXYLIN, NOVAMOX, SYNAMOX 250, 500 mg cap, 125 mg/5 ml dry syr; AMOXIL, MOX 250, 500 mg caps; 125 mg/5 ml dry syr; 250, 500 mg/vial inj. MOXYLONG : Amoxicillin 250 mg + probenecid 500 mg tab (also 500 mg + 500 mg DS tab).
11. **Amoxicillin + Cloxacillin:** NOVACLOX 250 + 250 mg cap, 125 + 125 mg pediatric tab, 125 + 125 mg inj, 250 + 250 mg inj, 500 + 500 mg inj.; 50 + 25 mg neonatal inj.
12. **Carbenicillin:** 1–2 g i.m. or 1–5 g i.v. 4–6 hourly; CARBELIN 1.0 g, 5.0 g per vial inj.
13. **Piperacillin:** 100–150 mg/kg/day in 3 divided doses (max 16 g/day) i.m. or i.v. The i.v. route is preferred when > 2 g is to be injected.
    PIPRAPEN 1 g, 2 g vials; PIPRACIL 2 g, 4 g vials for inj; contains 2 mEq Na^+ per g.
14. **Amoxicillin + Clavulanic acid (co-amoxiclav):** AUGMENTIN, ENHANCIN, AMONATE: Amoxicillin 250 mg + clavulanic acid 125 mg tab; 1–2 tab TDS, severe infections 4 tabs 6 hourly; CLAVAM 250 + 125 mg tab, 500 + 125 mg tab, 875 + 125 mg tab, 125 mg + 32 mg per 5 ml dry syr.
    Also AUGMENTIN, CLAVAM INJ; Amoxicillin 1 g + clavulanic acid 0.2 g vial and 0.5 g + 0.1 g vial; inject 1 vial deep i.m. or i.v. 6–8 hourly for severe infections.
15. **Ampicillin + Sulbactam:** SULBACIN, AMPITUM: Ampicillin 1 g + sulbactam 0.5 g per vial inj; 1–2 vial deep i.m. or i.v. injection 6–8 hourly.
16. **Sultamicillin tosylate (a complex salt of ampicillin and sulbactam):** BETAMPORAL, SULBACIN 375 mg tab.
17. **Piperacillin + Tazobactam:** 4 g + 0.5 g slow i.v. injection every 8 hours; PYBACTUM, TAZACT, TAZOBID, ZOSYN 4 g + 0.5 g per vial inj.

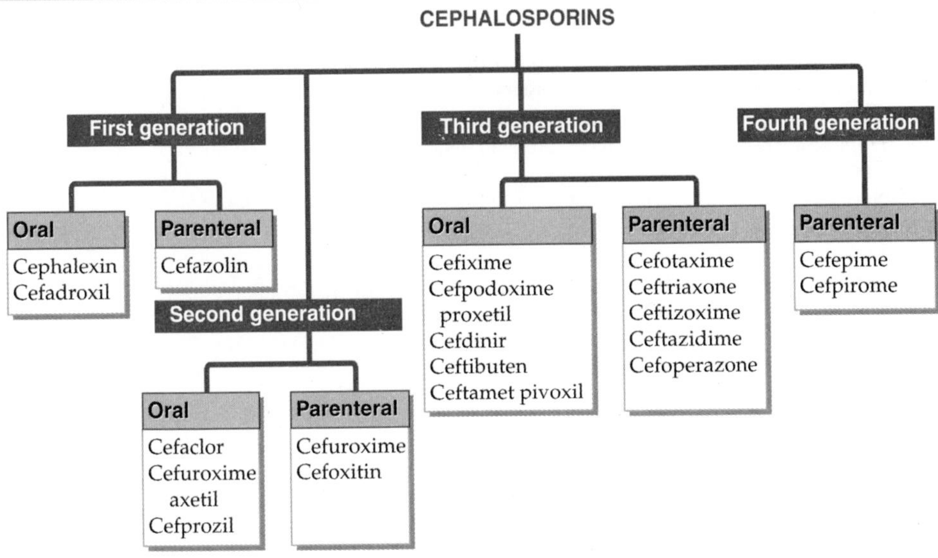
CEPHALOSPORINS
First generation
Oral
Cephalexin
Cefadroxil
Parenteral
Cefazolin
Second generation
Oral
Cefaclor
Cefuroxime axetil
Cefprozil
Parenteral
Cefuroxime
Cefoxitin
Third generation
Oral
Cefixime
Cefpodoxime proxetil
Cefdinir
Ceftibuten
Ceftamet pivoxil
Parenteral
Cefotaxime
Ceftriaxone
Ceftizoxime
Ceftazidime
Cefoperazone
Fourth generation
Parenteral
Cefepime
Cefpirome

Preparations

1. **Cefazolin:** 0.5 g 8 hourly (mild cases), 1 g 6 hourly (severe cases), children 25–50 mg/kg/day i.m. or i.v; for surgical prophylaxis 1.0 g half hour before surgery. ALCIZON, ORIZOLIN, REFLIN 0.25 g, 0.5 g, 1 g per vial inj.
2. **Cephalexin:** 0.25–1 g 6–8 hourly (children 25–100 mg/kg/day).
   CEPHACILLIN 250, 500 mg cap; SPORIDEX, ALCEPHIN, CEPHAXIN 250, 500 mg cap, 125 mg/5 ml dry syr., 100 mg/ml pediatric drops.
   ALCEPHIN-LA: Cephalexin + probenecid (250 + 250 mg and 500 + 500 mg) tabs.
3. **Cefadroxil:** 0.5–1 g BD. DROXYL 0.5, 1 g tab, 250 mg/5 ml syr; CEFADROX 0.5 g cap, 125 mg/5 ml syr and 250 mg kid tab; KEFLOXIN 0.5 g cap, 0.25 g distab, 125 mg/5 ml susp.
4. **Cefuroxime:** 0.75 –1.5 g i.m or i.v. 8 hourly, children 30–100 mg/kg/day;
   CEFOGEN, SUPACEF, FUROXIL 250 mg and 750 mg/vial inj.
5. **Cefuroxime axetil:** 250–500 mg BD oral, children half dose;
   CEFTUM, SPIZEF 125, 250, 500 mg captab and 125 mg/5 ml susp.
6. **Cefaclor:** 0.25–1.0 g 8 hourly oral; KEFLOR, VERCEF, DISTACLOR 250 mg cap, 125 and 250 mg distab, 125 mg/5 ml dry syr, 50 mg/ml ped. drops.
7. **Cefprozil:** 500 mg OD-BD (20 mg/kg/day); ORPROZIL 250, 500 mg tabs.
8. **Cefotaxime:** 1–2 g i.m./i.v. 6–12 hourly (children 50–100 mg/kg/day);
   OMNATAX, ORITAXIM, CLAFORAN 0.25, 0.5, 1.0 g per vial inj.
9. **Ceftizoxime:** 0.5–1 g i.m./i.v. 8 or 12 hourly; CEFIZOX, EPOCELIN 0.5 and 1 g per vial inj.
10. **Ceftriaxone:** Skin/soft tissue/urinary infections: 1–2 g i.v./i.m. per day;
    Meningitis: 4 g followed by 2 g i.v. (children 75–100 mg/kg) once daily for 7–10 days.
    Typhoid: 4 g i.v. daily × 2 days followed by 2 g/day (children 75 mg/kg) till 2 days after fever subsides.

OFRAMAX, MONOCEF, MONOTAX 0.25, 0.5, 1.0 g per vial inj.
Ceftriaxone 250 mg + Sulbactum 125 mg and 1 g + 500 mg: CEFTICHEK, SUPRAXONE vials for inj.
Ceftriaxone 1 g + Tazobactum 125 mg: EXTACEF-TAZO, FINECEF-T, MONTAZ vials for i.m./i.v. inj.

11. Ceftazidime: 0.5–2 g i.m. or i.v. every 8 hr, children 30 mg/kg/day. Resistant typhoid 30 mg/kg/day.
FORTUM, CEFAZID, ORZID 0.25, 0.5 and 1 g per vial inj.
12. Cefoperazone: 1–3 g i.m./i.v. 12 hourly; MAGNAMYCIN 0.25 g, 1, 2 g inj; CEFOMYCIN, NEGAPLUS 1 g inj.
Cefoperazone 500 mg + Sulbactum 500 mg: CEFOBETA, KEFBACTUM vial for inj, also CEFACTUM 1 g + 1 g vial for inj.
13. Cefixime: 200–400 mg BD; TOPCEF, ORFIX 100, 200 mg tab/cap, CEFSPAN 100 mg cap, 100 mg/5 ml syr, TAXIM-O 100, 200 mg tab, 50 mg/5ml dry syr.
14. Cefpodoxime proxetil: 200 mg BD (max 800 mg/day); CEFOPROX, CEPODEM, DOXCEF 100, 200 mg tab 50 mg/5 ml and 100 mg/5 ml dry syr.
15. Cefdinir: 300 mg BD: SEFDIN, ADCEF 300 mg cap, 125 mg/5 ml susp.
16. Ceftibuten: 200 mg BD or 400 mg OD; PROCADAX 400 mg cap, 90 mg/5 ml powder for oral suspension.
17. Ceftamet pivoxil: 500 mg TDS oral; ALTAMET 250 mg tab, CEPIME-O 500 mg tab.
18. Cefepime: 1–2 g (50 mg/kg) i.v. 8–12 hourly; KEFAGE, CEFICAD, CEPIME 0.5, 1.0 g inj.
19. Cefpirome: 1–2 g i.m./i.v. 12 hourly; CEFROM, CEFORTH 1.0 g inj., BACIROM, CEFOR 0.25, 0.5, 1.0 g inj.

Monobactam

Aztreonam: 0.5–2 g i.m. or i.v. 6–12 hourly; AZENAM, TREZAM 0.5, 1.0, 2.0 g per vial inj.

Carbapenems

1. Imipenem-cilastatin: 0.5 g i.v. 6 hourly (max 4 g/day). IMINEM 250 + 250 mg and 500 + 500 mg/vial inj., LASTINEM 125 + 125 mg, 250 + 250 mg, 500 + 500 mg and 1 g + 1 g per vial inj.

2. **Meropenem:** 0.5–2 g i.v. 8 hourly (10–20 mg/kg every 8 hours); MERONEM, UBPENEM 0.5, 1.0 g per vial inj.
3. **Faropenem:** 150–300 mg TDS oral; FARONEM, FAROZET 150, 200 mg tab.
4. **Doripenem:** 500 mg slow i.v. infusion over 1 hour every 8 hours; DORIGLEN 500 mg/vial inj., SUDOPEN 250, 500 mg/vial inj.

Aminoglycoside Antibiotics

Systemic aminoglycosides			Topical aminoglycosides	
Streptomycin	Gentamicin	Kanamycin	Neomycin	Framycetin
Tobramycin	Amikacin	Sisomicin		
Netilmicin	Paromomycin			

Preparations

1. **Streptomycin:** Acute infections: 1 g (0.75 g in those above 50 yr age) i.m. (15 mg/kg) BD for 7–10 days. Tuberculosis: 1 g or 0.75 g i.m. OD or thrice weekly for 30–60 days; AMBISTRYN-S 0.75, 1 g dry powder per vial for inj.
2. **Gentamicin:** 3–5 mg/kg/day i.m. in a single dose or divided in 8 hourly doses or in an i.v. line over 30–60 min (dose reduction needed in elderly and in renal insufficiency), 0.1–0.3% topically in eye or on skin. GARAMYCIN, GENTASPORIN, GENTICYN 20, 60, 80, 240 mg per vial inj; also 0.3% eye/ear drops, 0.1% skin cream.
3. **Kanamycin:** 0.5 g i.m. BD (15 mg/kg/day): KANAMYCIN, KANCIN, KANAMAC 0.5, 0.75, 1 g inj.
4. **Tobramycin:** 3–5 mg/kg/day i.m. in 1–3 doses; TOBACIN 20, 60, 80 mg in 2 ml inj. 0.3% eye drops. TOBRANEG 20, 40, 80 mg per 2 ml inj., TOBRABACT 0.3% eye drops.
5. **Amikacin:** 15 mg/kg/day i.m. in 1–3 doses; urinary tract infection 7.5 mg/kg/day; AMICIN, MIKACIN, MIKAJECT 100 mg, 250 mg, 500 mg in 2 ml inj.

6. **Sisomicin:** 3–5 mg/kg/day i.m.; ENSAMYCIN, SISOPTIN 50 mg, 10 mg (pediatric) per ml in 1 ml amps.
7. **Netilmicin:** 4–6 mg/kg/day i.m. in 1–3 doses; NETROMYCIN 10, 25, 50 mg in 1 ml, 200 mg in 2 ml and 300 mg in 3 ml inj., NETICIN 200 mg (2 ml), 300 mg (3 ml) inj.
8. **Neomycin:** 0.25–1 g QID oral, 0.3–0.5% topical.
   NEOMYCIN SULPHATE 350, 500 mg tab, 0.3% skin oint, 0.5% skin cream, eye oint.
   NEBASULF: Neomycin sulph. 5 mg, bacitracin 250 U, sulfacetamide 60 mg/g oint. and powder for surface application.
   POLYBIOTIC CREAM: Neomycin sulph. 5 mg, polymyxin 5,000 IU, gramicidin 0.25 mg/g cream.
   NEOSPORIN: Neomycin 3400 iu, polymyxin B 5000 iu, bacitracin 400 iu/g oint; NEOSPORIN-H: Neomycin 3400 iu, polymyxin B 10000 iu, hydrocortisone 10 mg per ml ear drops.
9. **Framycetin:** 0.5%–1.0% topically in eye or on skin;
   SOFRAMYCIN, FRAMYGEN 1% skin cream, 0.5% eye drops or oint.
10. **Paromomycin:** *Oral*: 500 mg TDS (25–30 mg/kg/day) for amoebiasis, giardiasis, etc.
    Intramuscular: 15 mg (11 mg base) per kg/day for 21 days for Kala-azar.

Tetracyclines

1. **Oxytetracycline:** 250–500 mg TDS–QID oral, 500 mg 6–12 hourly by slow i.v. inj; 1–3% by topical application;
   TERRAMYCIN 250, 500 mg cap, 50 mg/ml in 10 ml vials inj; 3% skin oint, 1% eye/ear oint.
2. **Tetracycline:** 250–500 mg TDS–QID oral; 1–3% topically in eye/ear/on skin;
   ACHROMYCIN, HOSTACYCLINE, RESTECLIN 250, 500 mg cap, 3% skin oint, 1% eye/ear drops and oint.
3. **Demeclocycline (Demethylchlortetracycline):** 300–600 mg BD oral; LEDERMYCIN 150, 300 mg cap/tab.
4. **Doxycycline:** 200 mg initially followed by 100–200 mg OD oral;
   TETRADOX, DOXICIP, DOXT, NOVADOX 100 mg cap.
5. **Minocycline:** 100 mg OD–BD oral; CYANOMYCIN, CNN 50, 100 mg caps.

6. Tigecycline: 100 mg loading dose, followed by 50 mg 12 hourly i.v. infusion over 30–60 min for 5–14 days. TYGACIL, TEVRAN, TIGIMAX 50 mg lyophilized powder/vial inj.

Chloramphenicol

1. Chloramphenicol: 250–500 mg 6 hourly oral (max 28 g total in a course), children 25–50 mg/kg/day; 0.5–1% topically in eye, 5–10% topically in ear; rarely 1% on skin;
   CHLOROMYCETIN, ENTEROMYCETIN, PARAXIN, 250 mg, 500 mg cap, 1% eye oint, 0.5% eye drops, 5% ear drops, 1% applicaps, VANMYCETIN 0.4% eye drops, 250 mg opticaps, LYKACETIN 1% skin cream, 10% otic solution, OCUCHLOR 0.5% eye drops.
2. Chloramphenicol palmitate (tasteless insoluble ester of chloramphenicol for liquid oral formulation): CHLOROMYCETIN PALMITATE, ENTEROMYCETIN, PARAXIN 125 mg/5 ml oral susp.
3. Chloramphenicol succinate (soluble ester of chloramphenicol for i.v. injection): ENTEROMYCETIN, CHLOROMYCETIN SUCCINATE, KEMICETINE 1 g/vial inj, PHENIMYCIN 0.25, 0.5, 1.0 g inj.

Macrolide Antibiotics

1. Erythromycin: 250–500 mg 6 hourly (max. 4 g/day), children 30–60 mg/kg/day.
   (a) Erythromycin (base): ERYSAFE 250 mg tabs, EROMED 333 mg tab, 125 mg/5 ml susp, 2% lotion, 4% gel.
   (b) Erythromycin stearate: ERYTHROCIN 250, 500 mg tab, 100 mg/5 ml susp., 100 mg/ml ped. drops. ETROCIN, ERYSTER 250 mg tab, 100 mg/5 ml dry syr.
   (c) Erythromycin estolate (lauryl sulfate): ALTHROCIN 250, 500 mg tab, 125 mg kid tab, 125 mg/5 ml and 250 mg/5 ml dry syr, 100 mg/ml ped. drops, E-MYCIN 100, 250 mg tab, 100 mg/5 ml dry syr; EMTHROCIN 250 mg tab, 125 mg/5 ml dry syr.

(d) **Erythromycin ethylsuccinate:** ERYNATE 100 mg/5 ml dry syr, ERYTHROCIN 100 mg/ml drops, 125 mg/5 ml syr.

2. **Roxithromycin:** 150–300 mg BD 30 min before meals, children 2.5–5 mg/kg BD; ROXID, ROXIBID, RULIDE 150, 300 mg tab, 50 mg kid tab, 50 mg/5 ml liquid; ROXEM 50 mg kid tab, 150 mg tab.
3. **Clarithromycin:** 250 mg BD for 7 days; severe cases 500 mg BD upto 14 days; CLARIBID 250, 500 mg tab, 250 mg/5 ml dry syr; CLARIMAC 250, 500 mg tabs; SYNCLAR 250 mg tab, 125 mg/5 ml dry syr.
4. **Azithromycin:** 500 mg once daily 1 hour before or 2 hours after food (children above 6 month 10 mg/kg) for 3 days is sufficient for most infections; AZITHRAL 250, 500 mg cap and 250 mg per 5 ml dry syr; AZIWOK 250 mg cap, 100 mg kid tab, 100 mg/5 ml and 200 mg/5 ml susp. AZIWIN 100, 250, 500 mg tab, 200 mg/5 ml liq. Also AZITHRAL 500 mg inj. for i.m. use.
5. **Spiramycin:** 3 million units (MU) twice daily oral; ROVAMYCIN 1.5 MU, 3 MU tabs, 0.375 MU/5 ml susp.

Lincosamide Antibiotics

1. **Lincomycin:** 500 mg TDS–QID oral; 600 mg i.m. or by i.v. infusion 6–12 hrly; LINCOCIN 500 mg cap, 600 mg/2 ml inj; LYNX 250, 500 mg cap, 125 mg/5 ml syr, 300 mg/ml inj in 1, 2 ml amp.
2. **Clindamycin:** 150–300 mg (Children 3–6 mg/kg) QID oral; 200–600 mg i.v. 8 hourly; DALCAP 150 mg cap; CLINCIN 150, 300 mg cap; DALCIN, DALCINEX 150, 300 mg cap, 300 mg/2 ml and 600 mg/4 ml inj. ACNESOL, CLINDAC-A 1% topical solution and gel for acne vulgaris.

Aminocyclitol Antibiotic

1. **Spectinomycin:** Gonorrhoea—2 g i.m. single dose (4 g in resistant cases); disseminated gonococcal infection—2 g i.m. BD. MYSPEC, TROBICIN 2 g vial for i.m. inj.

Glycopeptide Antibiotics

1. **Vancomycin:** 125–500 mg oral, 0.5 g 6 hourly or 1.0 g 12 hourly by i.v. infusion over 1 hour; VANCOCIN-CP; VANCOGEN, VANCORID-CP 500 mg/vial inj; VANCOLED 0.5, 1.0 g inj, VANCOMYCIN 500 mg tab, 250 mg cap, 500 mg/vial inj.
2. **Teicoplanin:** 400 mg first day—then 200 mg daily i.v. or i.m.; severe infection 400 mg 12 hourly × 3 doses—then 400 mg daily; TARGOCID, TECOPLAN, TECOCIN 200, 400 mg per vial inj. for reconstitution.

Oxazolidinone

1. **Linezolid:** 600 mg BD, oral/i.v.; LIZOLID, LINOSPAN 600 mg tab; LINOX, LINOSPAN 600 mg tab, 600 mg/300 ml i.v. infusion.

Polypeptide Antibiotics

1. **Polymyxin B:** 5000–10,000 U/g for topical application (1 mg=10,000 U); NEOSPORIN POWDER: 5000 U with neomycin sulf. 3400 U and bacitracin 400 U per g. NEOSPORIN EYE DROPS: 5000 U with neomycin sulf. 1700 U and gramicidin 0.25 mg per ml. NEOSPORIN-H EAR DROPS: 10,000 U with neomycin sulf. 3400 U and hydrocortisone 10 mg per ml.
2. **Colistin sulfate:** 25–100 mg TDS oral; WALAMYCIN 12.5 mg (25000 i.u.) per 5 ml dry syr, COLISTOP 12.5 mg/5 ml and 25 mg/5 ml dry syr.
3. **Bacitracin:** 250–500 U/g for topical application (1 U = 26 μg); In NEBASULF: bacitracin 250 U+ neomycin + sulfacetamide 60 mg/g powder, skin oint, eye oint; in NEOSPORIN 400 U/g powder.

Urinary Antiseptics

1. **Nitrofurantoin:** 50–100 mg 3 to 4 times a day oral; FURADANTIN 50, 100 mg tab, 25 mg/5 ml susp, URINIF 100 mg tab.
2. **Methenamine (Hexamine) mandelate:** 1.0 g 3–4 times/day oral; MANDELAMINE 0.5 g, 1.0 g tabs.
3. **Nalidixic acid:** 0.5–1 g TDS–QID oral (*See p.* 133)

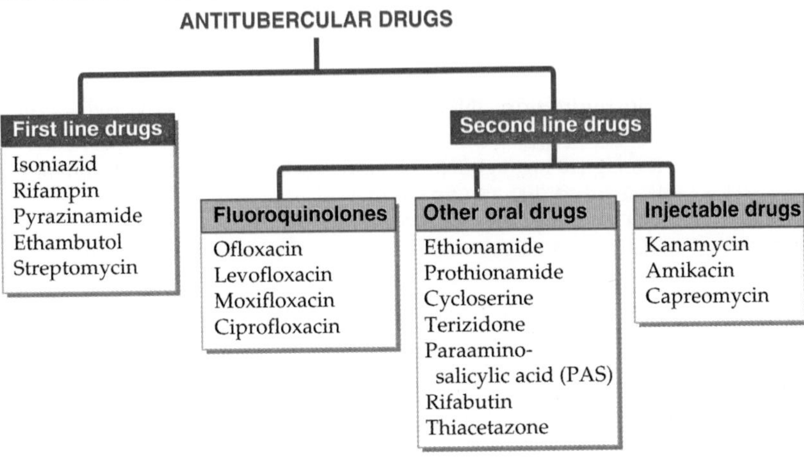
ANTITUBERCULAR DRUGS
First line drugs
Isoniazid
Rifampin
Pyrazinamide
Ethambutol
Streptomycin
Second line drugs
Fluoroquinolones
Ofloxacin
Levofloxacin
Moxifloxacin
Ciprofloxacin
Other oral drugs
Ethionamide
Prothionamide
Cycloserine
Terizidone
Paraamino-salicylic acid (PAS)
Rifabutin
Thiacetazone
Injectable drugs
Kanamycin
Amikacin
Capreomycin

Preparations

Antitubercular Drugs

1. **Isoniazid (Isonicotinic acid hydrazide, INH):** 300 mg (5 mg/kg) daily or 600–900 mg (10 mg/kg) thrice weekly oral; ISONEX 100, 300 mg tabs, ISOKIN 100 mg tab, 100 mg per 5 ml liq.
2. **Rifampin (Rifampicin):** 600 mg (10 mg/kg) daily or thrice weekly oral one hour before or two hours after meals; RCIN 150, 300, 450, 600 mg caps, 100 mg/5 ml susp. RIMACTANE, RIMPIN 150, 300, 450 mg caps, 100 mg/5 ml syr; RIFAMYCIN 450 mg cap, ZUCOX 300, 450, 600 mg tabs.
3. **Pyrazinamide:** 25 mg/kg daily or 35 mg/kg thrice weekly oral; PYZINA 0.5, 0.75, 1.0 g tabs, 0.3 g kid tab; PZA-CIBA 0.5, 0.75 g tabs, 250 mg/5 ml syr; RIZAP 0.75, 1.0 g tabs.
4. **Ethambutol:** 15 mg/kg daily or 30 mg/kg thrice weekly oral; MYCOBUTOL, MYAMBUTOL, COMBUTOL 0.2, 0.4, 0.6, 0.8, 1.0 g tabs.
5. **Streptomycin:** 1000 mg (15 mg/kg) daily or thrice weekly i.m.; patients over 60 years age—reduce dose to 10 mg/kg or 500–750 mg/day i.m. AMBISTRYN-S 0.75 g and 1.0 g dry powder per vial for i.m. inj.
6. **Paraaminosalicylic acid (PAS):** 10–12 g (200 mg/kg) per day oral in divided doses; SODIUM-PAS 0.5 g tab, 80 g/100g granules.
7. **Ethionamide:** 0.5–0.75 g (10–15 mg/kg) per day oral; ETHIDE, ETHIOCID, MYOBID 250 mg tab.
8. **Prothionamide:** 0.5–0.75 g (10–15 mg/kg/day) oral; PROTHICID, PETHIDE 250 mg tab.
9. **Cycloserine:** 250 mg BD, increased if tolerated upto 750 mg per day oral; CYCLORINE, COXERIN, MYSER 250 mg cap.
10. **Terizidone:** 500–700 mg/day oral; TERICOX 250 mg cap.
11. **Kanamycin:** 0.75–1.0 g/day (10–15 mg/kg/day) i.m.; KANCIN, KANAMAC 0.5, 1 g inj.

ALTERNATIVE CLASSIFICATION

ANTITUBERCULAR DRUGS

Group I First line oral drugs	Group II Injectable drugs	Group III Fluoroquinolones	Group IV Second line oral drugs	Group V Unclear efficacy drugs
Isoniazid	Streptomycin	Ofloxacin	Ethionamide	Thiacetazone
Rifampin	Kanamycin	Levofloxacin	Prothionamide	Clarithromycin
Pyrazinamide	Amikacin	Moxifloxacin	Cycloserine	Clofazimine
Ethambutol	Capreomycin	Ciprofloxacin	Terizidone	Linezolid
			Para amino-salicylic acid	

ANTILEPROTIC DRUGS

Sulfone	Phenazine derivative	Antitubercular drugs	Other antibiotics
Dapsone	Clofazimine	Rifampin	Ofloxacin
		Ethionamide	Moxifloxacin
			Minocycline
			Clarithromycin

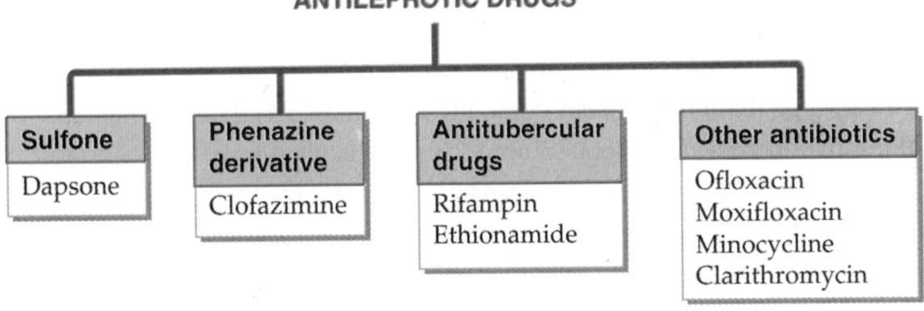

12. **Amikacin:** 0.75–1.0 g (15 mg/kg) i.m. daily; AMICIN, MIKACIN, MIKAJECT 250 mg, 500 mg inj.
13. **Capreomycin:** 0.75–1.0 g (15 mg/kg) i.m. daily; KAPOCIN 0.5 g, 0.75 g, 1.0 g inj, CAPREOTEC 1.0g inj.
14. **Ciprofloxacin:** 750 mg BD oral.
15. **Ofloxacin:** 800 mg OD oral.
16. **Levofloxacin:** 750 mg OD.
17. **Moxifloxacin:** 400 mg OD.
18. **Rifabutin:** 300 mg (5 mg/kg) OD oral; RIBUTIN 150 mg tab.

Some antitubercular combinations

RIFATER: Rifampin 120 mg, isoniazid 80 mg, pyrazinamide 250 mg tab.

R-CINEX: Rifampin 600 mg, isoniazid 300 mg tab; R-CINEX-Z: Rifampin 225 mg, isoniazid 150 mg, pyrazinamide 750 mg tab. RIMACTAZID, RIFADIN-INH, Rifampin 450 mg, isoniazid 300 mg tab.

MYCONEX 600 and 800; Isoniazid 300 mg, ethambutol 600 mg or 800 mg tab, COMBUNEX Isoniazid 300 mg, ethambutol 800 mg tab.

ARZIDE, ISORIFAM: Rifampin 450 mg, isoniazid 300 mg cap.

BI-TEBEN, ISOZONE: Isoniazid 75 mg, thiacetazone 37.5 mg tab, ISOZONE FORTE—double strength.

UNITHIBEN Isoniazid 75 mg, thiacetazone 37.5 mg tab.

INAPAS: sod PAS 834 mg, isoniazid 25 mg tab; sod PAS 3.34 g + isoniazid 100 mg per measure granules.

INABUTOL: Isoniazid 150 mg, ethambutol 400 mg tab; INABUTOL FORTE—double strength.

ISOKIN–300: Isoniazid 300 mg, vit B_6 10 mg tab.

IPCAZIDE: Isoniazid 100 mg, vit B_6 5 mg per 5 ml liq.

Antitubercular Combipacks (packs of 1 day's dose)

AKT-4: R 450 mg 1 cap + Z 750 mg 2 tab + E 800 mg + H 300 mg 1 tab.
AKT-3: R 450 mg 1 cap + E 800 mg + H 300 mg 1 tab.
CX-5: R 450 mg 1 cap + Z 750 mg 2 tab + E800 mg + H 300 mg + pyridoxine 10 mg 1 tab.
RIFACOM-Z and RIMACTAZID-Z: R 450 mg + H 300 mg 1 tab. + Z 750 mg 2 tab.
RIFACOM-EZ: R 450 mg + H 300 mg 1 tab. + Z 750 mg 2 tab + E 800 mg 1 tab.

Note: *See* Index for preparations of ciprofloxacin, ofloxacin, levofloxacin and moxifloxacin.

Antileprotic Drugs

1. Dapsone (Diaminodiphenyl sulfone, DDS): 100 mg/day; DAPSONE 25, 50, 100 mg tab.
2. Clofazimine: 50 mg daily + 300 mg once a month; CLOFOZINE, HANSEPRAN 50, 100 mg caps.
3. Rifampin: 600 mg once a month
4. Ethionamide: 250 mg/day oral
5. Ofloxacin: 400 mg/day oral
6. Moxifloxacin: 400 mg/day oral
7. Minocycline: 100 mg/day oral
8. Clarithromycin: 500 mg/day oral.

Note: See Index for preparations of other drugs.

For erythema nodosum leprosum (type 2)

Thalidomide: 100–300 mg OD at bed time; THAANGIO 100 mg, THALODA 50, 100 mg cap.
(For multiple myeloma—200 mg OD; max 800 mg/day)

12 Antifungal, Antiviral, Antiprotozoal and Anthelmintic Drugs

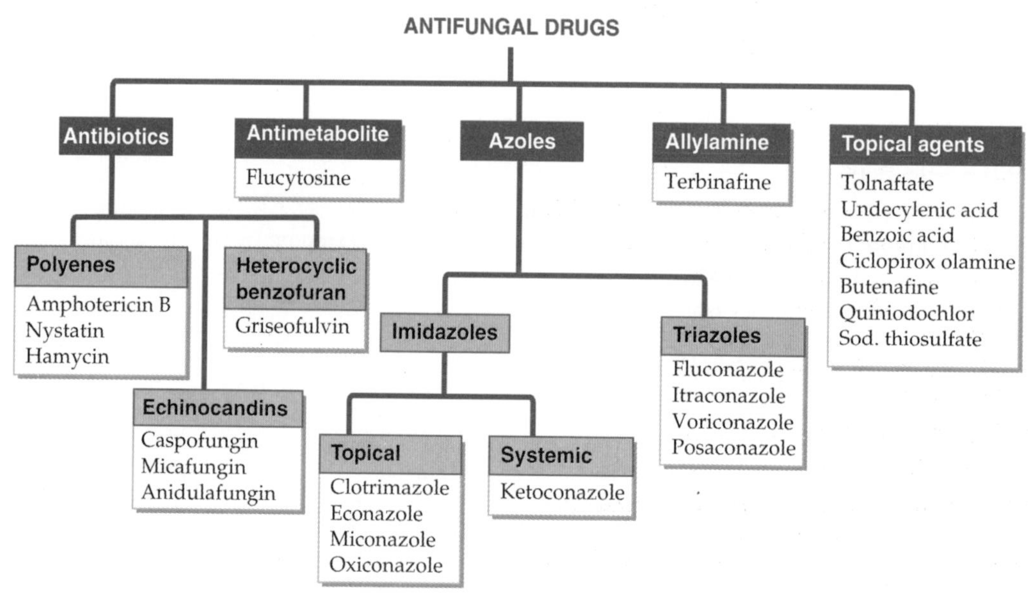

Preparations

1. **Amphotericin B:** 0.3–0.7 mg/kg daily by slow i.v. infusion over 4–8 hours (total dose 3–4 g); 0.5 mg intrathecal, 3% topically in ear, 50–100 mg QID oral; FUNGIZONE INTRAVENOUS, MYCOL 50 mg dry powder per vial for i.v. infusion, FUNGIZONE OTIC 3% ear drops.

   Liposomal amphotericin B: 3-5 mg/kg/day i.v. infusion; FUNGISOME 10 mg, 25 mg, 50 mg per vial inj, AMPHOLIP 10 mg/2 ml, 50 mg/10 ml, 100 mg/20 ml inj.
2. **Nystatin:** 5 lac U 8 hourly oral, 1 lac U nightly for vaginal insertion, 10,000 U/ml for buccal application; 1 lac U per g for application over skin and in the eye;
   MYCOSTATIN 5 lac U tab, 1 lac U vaginal tab, 1 lac U/g oint, NYSTIN EYE 1 lac U/g ophthalmic oint.
3. **Hamycin:** 2–5 lac U/g for topical application, 4 lac U vaginal application;
   HAMYCIN 5 lac U/g oint, 2 lac U/ml susp for topical use, 4 lac U vaginal ovules.
4. **Caspofungin:** 70 mg infused i.v. over 1 hour (loading dose), followed by 50 mg i.v. daily.
   CANCIDAS 70 mg in 10 ml and 50 mg in 10 ml inj.
5. **Griseofulvin:** 125–250 mg QID oral taken with meals; GRISOVIN–FP, GRISORAL, WALAVIN-FP 250 mg tab.
6. **Clotrimazole:** 1% topical application twice daily, 100 mg intravaginal at bed time:
   SURFAZ, CLODERM 1% lotion, cream, powder; 100 mg vaginal tab. CANDID 1% cream, mouth paint.
7. **Econazole:** 1% topical application 2–3 times daily, 150 mg intravaginal every night;
   ECONAZOLE 1% oint, 150 mg vaginal tab; ECODERM 1% cream.
8. **Miconazole:** 2% topical application 2–3 times daily, 100 mg intravaginal nightly;
   DAKTARIN 2% gel, 2% powder and solution; GYNODAKTARIN 2% vaginal gel; ZOLE 2% oint, lotion, dusting powder and spray, 1% ear drops, 100 mg vaginal ovules.
9. **Oxiconazole:** 1% topical; OXIZON, ZODERM 1% + benzoic acid 0.25% cream and lotion.

10. **Ketoconazole:** 200 mg OD–BD oral, 2% topical application; FUNGICIDE, NIZRAL, FUNAZOLE, KETOVATE 200 mg tab, FUNGINOC, NIZRAL 2% oint, 2% shampoo (for dandruff), KETOVATE 2% cream, DANRUF 2% shampoo, HYPHORAL 2% lotion.
11. **Fluconazole:** For tinea infections, cutaneous and vaginal candidiasis 150 mg oral weekly; for systemic mycosis 200–400 mg daily oral/i.v., for fungal keratitis 0.3% topically in eye; SYSCAN, ZOCON, FORCAN, FLUZON 50, 100, 150, 200 mg caps, 200 mg/100 ml i.v. infusion, SYSCAN 0.3% eye drops.
12. **Itraconazole:** 200 mg OD–BD oral (for systemic mycosis), 200 mg OD oral for vaginal candidiasis and dermatophytosis; SPORANOX, CANDITRAL, FLUCOVER 100 mg cap, ITASPOR 100 mg cap, 200 mg/20 ml vial.
13. **Voriconazole:** Oral–200 mg BD taken 1 hour before or 1 hour after meal; Intravenous—initially 6 mg/kg 12 hourly 2 doses, then 3-4 mg/kg 12 hourly. Drug is to be reconstituted and diluted, infused at not more than 3 mg/kg/hr. VFEND 50 mg, 200 mg tabs, 40 mg/ml oral susp; 200 mg vial for i.v. infusion; FUNGIVOR 200 mg tab.
14. **Posaconazole:** 200 mg 4 times a day or 400 mg twice a day with meals. NOXAFIL 200 mg/5 ml susp.
15. **Terbinafine:** 250 mg OD oral, 1% topical application; LAMISIL, SEBIFIN, DASKIL 250 mg tab, 1% topical cream. EXIFINE 125, 250 mg tabs, 1% cream, TERBIDERM 1% cream.
16. **Tolnaftate:** 1% topical application; TINADERM, TINAVATE 1% lotion, TOLNADERM 1% cream.
17. **Ciclopirox olamine:** 1% topical and vaginal application; BATRAFEN 1% cream, 1% topical solution, 1% vaginal cream, OLAMIN 1% cream.
18. **Undecylenic acid:** 5–10% topical application; TINEAFAX: Zinc undecenoate 8% zinc naphthenate 8%, mesulphen 8%, methyl salicylate 2.5%, terpineol 2.5% oint.
19. **Benzoic acid:** 5% topical application; RINGCUTTER 5% benzoic acid + 3% salicylic acid oint.
20. **Quiniodochlor:** 3–10% topical application; VIOFORM 3% cream, DERMOQUINOL 4%, 8% cream.
21. **Butenafine:** 1% topical; BUTOP, FINTOP 1% cream.
22. **Sodium thiosulfate:** 20% topical application; in KARPIN LOTION 20% lotion.

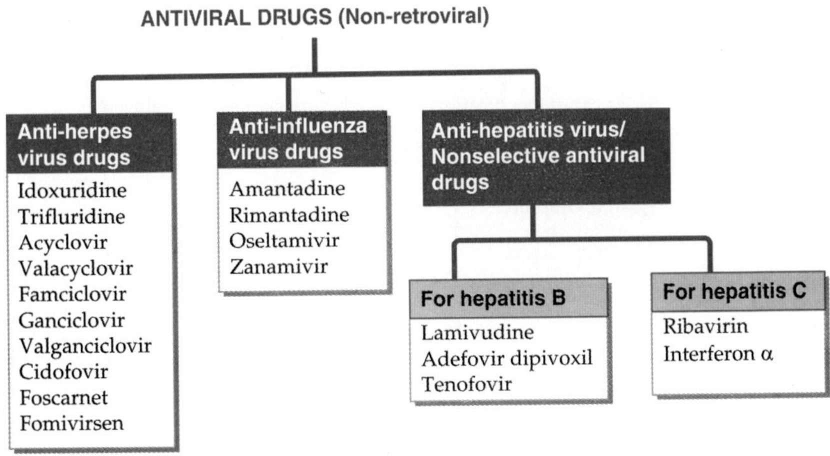
ANTIVIRAL DRUGS (Non-retroviral)
Anti-herpes virus drugs
Idoxuridine
Trifluridine
Acyclovir
Valacyclovir
Famciclovir
Ganciclovir
Valganciclovir
Cidofovir
Foscarnet
Fomivirsen
Anti-influenza virus drugs
Amantadine
Rimantadine
Oseltamivir
Zanamivir
Anti-hepatitis virus/ Nonselective antiviral drugs
For hepatitis B
Lamivudine
Adefovir dipivoxil
Tenofovir
For hepatitis C
Ribavirin
Interferon α

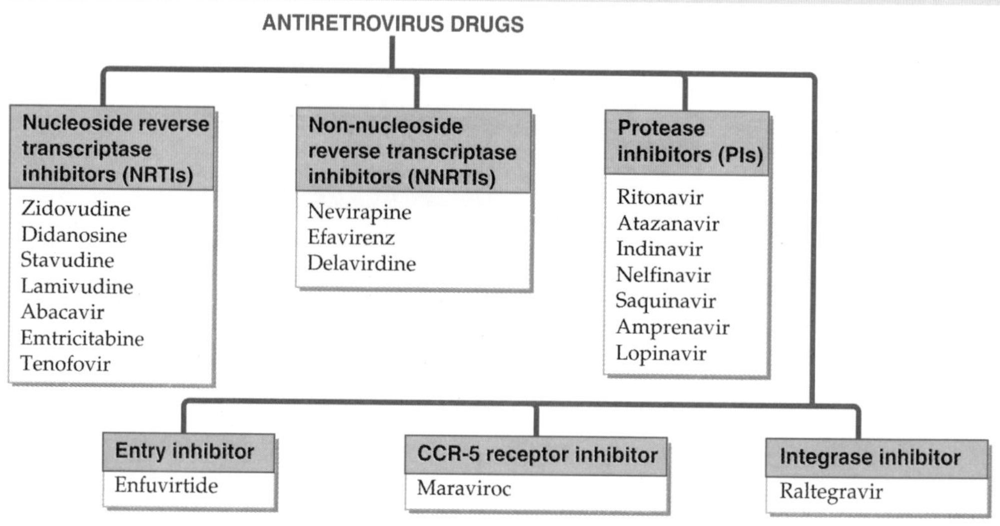
ANTIRETROVIRUS DRUGS
Nucleoside reverse transcriptase inhibitors (NRTIs)
Zidovudine
Didanosine
Stavudine
Lamivudine
Abacavir
Emtricitabine
Tenofovir
Non-nucleoside reverse transcriptase inhibitors (NNRTIs)
Nevirapine
Efavirenz
Delavirdine
Protease inhibitors (PIs)
Ritonavir
Atazanavir
Indinavir
Nelfinavir
Saquinavir
Amprenavir
Lopinavir
Entry inhibitor
Enfuvirtide
CCR-5 receptor inhibitor
Maraviroc
Integrase inhibitor
Raltegravir

Preparations

Antiviral Drugs (Non-retroviral)

1. **Idoxuridine:** 0.1% topically in eye 1 hourly to 6 hourly, apply 0.1% eye ointment at night; IDURIN, TOXIL 0.1% eye drops and oint.
2. **Acyclovir:** 200 mg 5 times a day oral (15 mg/kg/day), 5–10 mg/kg 8 hourly by slow i.v. infusion, 5% topical application 6 times a day; ZOVIRAX 200 mg tab, 250 mg/vial for i.v. inj; CYCLOVIR 200 mg tab, 5% skin cream; HERPEX 200 mg tab, 3% eye oint, 5% skin cream; OCUVIR 200, 400, 800 mg tab, 3% eye oint, ACIVIR-DT 200, 400, 800 mg tab. ACIVIR EYE 3% oint.
3. **Valacyclovir:** For genital herpes simplex 0.5-1.0 g BD × 10 days, suppressive treatment 0.5 g OD × 6–12 months.
   For orolabial herpes 2 g BD × 1 day
   For herpes zoster 1 g TDS × 7 days.
   VALCIVIR 0.5 g, 1.0 g tabs.
4. **Famciclovir:** Genital herpes (1st episode) 250 mg TDS × 5 days; recurrent cases 250 mg BD for upto 1 year. Herpes zoster and orolabial herpes 500 mg TDS for 7–10 days. FAMTREX 250, 500 mg tabs.
5. **Ganciclovir:** For treatment and prophylaxis of CMV infections—5 mg/kg BD initially, followed by OD; GANGUARD 250, 500 mg tabs.
6. **Amantadine:** 100 mg BD, elderly—half dose, children 5 mg/kg/day; AMANTREL, NEAMAN 100 mg tab.
7. **Rimantadine:** 100 mg BD, elderly 100 mg OD, child 5 mg/kg/day; FLUMADINE 100 mg tab, 50 mg/5 ml syr.
8. **Oseltamivir:** therapeutic dose—75 mg BD × 5 days; prophylactic dose—75 mg OD; TAMIFLU, ANTIFLU 75 mg cap, 12 mg/ml susp, FLUVIR 75 mg cap.

9. **Zanamivir:** therapeutic dose—10 mg BD by inhalation; prophylactic dose—10 mg OD; RELENZA 5 mg per actuation powder inhaler.
10. **Adefovir dipivoxil:** 10 mg/day oral; ADESERA, ADFOVIR 10 mg tab.
11. **Tenofovir:** 300 mg OD; TENOF, TENTIDE 300 mg tab.
12. **Ribavirin:** 200 mg QID (children 10 mg/kg/day); VIRAZIDE, RIBAVIN 100, 200 mg caps, 50 mg/5 ml syr.
13. **Interferon α_{2A}:** 2.5–5 MU/m² s.c. or i.m. 3 times per week; ALFERON 3MU/vial inj.
14. **Interferon α_{2B}:** 3–10 MU s.c. or i.m. thrice weekly; REALFA-2B, SHANFERON, VIRAFERON 3MU, 5MU vials for inj.

Antiretroviral Drugs

15. **Zidovudine (Azidothymidine, AZT):** Adults 300 mg BD; Children 180 mg/m² (max 200 mg) BD.

    RETROVIR, ZIDOVIR 100 mg cap 300 mg tab, 50 mg/5 ml syr, ZIDOMAX, ZYDOWIN 100 mg cap, 300 mg tab (to be taken with plenty of water).
16. **Didanosine:** 400 mg/day (for $\geq$ 60 kg BW), 250 mg/day ($<$ 50 kg BW); 1 hour before or 2 hours after meals; DINEX EC, DD RETRO, VIROSINE DR 250, 400 mg tabs.
17. **Stavudine:** 30 mg BD; STAG, STAVIR, VIROSTAV 30, 40 mg caps.
18. **Lamivudine:** *For chronic hepatitis B*—100 mg OD;

    For HIV infection—150 mg BD (along with other antiretroviral drugs); LAMIVIR 150 mg tab, 150 mg/5 ml soln; LAMIVIR-HBV 100 mg tab; HEPTAVIR, LAMIDAC, LAMUVID 100, 150 mg tabs.
19. **Abacavir:** 300 mg BD or 600 mg OD (along with other antiretroviral drugs); ABAMUNE, ABAVIR 300 mg tab.
20. **Nevirapine:** 200 mg/day oral to be increased after 2 weeks to 200 mg BD; NEVIMUNE, NEVIVIR, NEVIPAN, NEVIRETRO 200 mg.

21. **Efavirenz:** 600 mg OD on empty stomach; EFFERVEN, VIRANZ, EVIRENZ, 200 mg cap, 600 mg tab.
22. **Atazanavir:** 300 mg OD with ritonavir 100 mg taken at meal time; ATAZOR 100, 150, 200, 300 mg caps.
23. **Indinavir:** 800 mg TDS; INDIVAN, INDIVIR, VIRODIN 400 mg cap.
24. **Nelfinavir:** 750 mg TDS; NELFIN, NELVIR, NEIVEX 250 mg tab.
25. **Ritonavir:** 600 mg BD to be taken with meal; RITOVIR 250 mg tab, RITOMUNE, RITOMAX 100 mg cap.
26. **Saquinavir:** 1200 mg TDS oral taken with or just after a meal or 1000 mg BD along with ritonavir 100 mg; SAQUIN 200 mg cap.
27. **Lopinavir:** 400 mg (taken with ritonavir 100 mg) BD with food.
    RITOMAX-L, V-LETRA: Lopinavir 133.3 mg + Ritonavir 33.3 mg cap.

Some Antiretroviral Combinations

1. **Lamivudine** 150 mg + **Zidovudine** 300 mg tab (1 tab BD);
   COMBIVIR, CYTOCOM, DUOVIR, LAMUZID, ZIDOLAM tab.
2. **Lamivudine** 150 mg + **Stavudine** 30 mg or 40 mg tab (1 tab BD);
   LAMIVIR-S, LAMOSTAD, VIROLIS tab.
3. **Lamivudine** 150 mg + **Zidovudine** 300 mg + **Nevirapine** 200 mg tab (1 tab BD);
   DUOVIR-N, CYTOCOM-N, NEXIVIR-Z.
4. **Lamivudine** 150 mg + **Stavudine** 30 mg or 40 mg + **Nevirapine** 200 mg tab (1 tab BD);
   LAMOSTAD-N, TROMUNE, VIROLANS.
5. **Lamivudine** 150 mg + **Zidovudine** 300 mg 2 tab and **Efavirenz** 600 mg 1 tab kit;
   CYTOCOM-E kit.

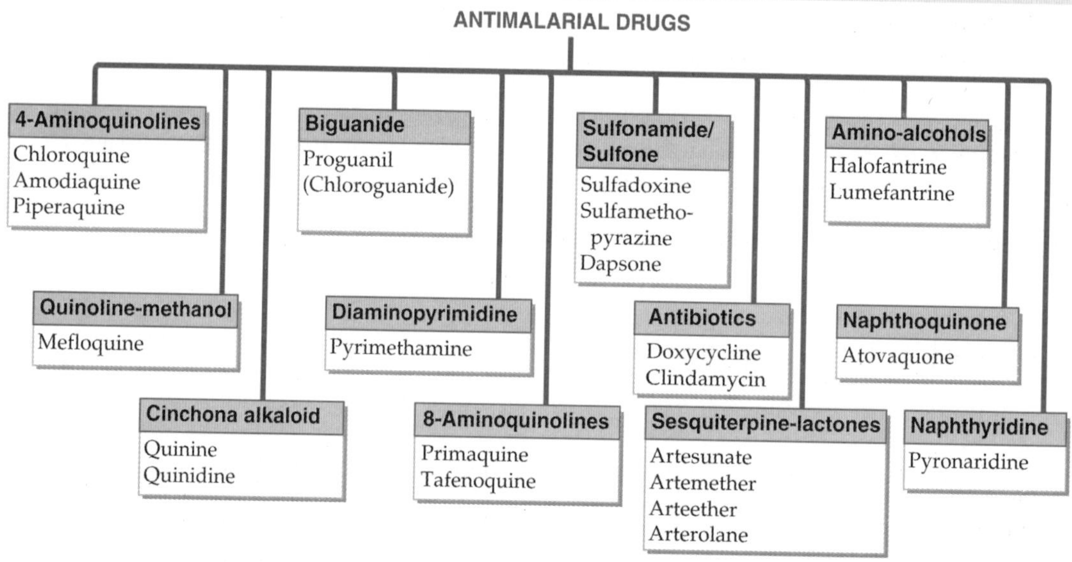
ANTIMALARIAL DRUGS
4-Aminoquinolines
Chloroquine
Amodiaquine
Piperaquine
Quinoline-methanol
Mefloquine
Cinchona alkaloid
Quinine
Quinidine
Biguanide
Proguanil
(Chloroguanide)
Diaminopyrimidine
Pyrimethamine
8-Aminoquinolines
Primaquine
Tafenoquine
Sulfonamide/
Sulfone
Sulfadoxine
Sulfametho-
pyrazine
Dapsone
Antibiotics
Doxycycline
Clindamycin
Sesquiterpine-lactones
Artesunate
Artemether
Arteether
Arterolane
Amino-alcohols
Halofantrine
Lumefantrine
Naphthoquinone
Atovaquone
Naphthyridine
Pyronaridine

Preparations

1. **Chloroquine:** For clinical cure: 600 mg (base) followed by 300 mg after 8 hours and 300 mg daily for 2 days (total 1500 mg); total dose (in 3 days) for infants 150 mg, children 1–4 years 200–400 mg, 5–10 years 600–1000 mg. For suppressive prophylaxis: 300 mg weekly (only in chloroquine sensitive *P. falciparum* areas).
   Chloroquine phosphate: (250 mg = 150 mg base): RESOCHIN 150 mg (base) tab; CLOQUIN, LARIAGO, NIVAQUIN-P 250 mg tab, 500 mg forte tab, 100 mg (base) per 10 ml oral susp., 40 mg (base)/ml inj in 2 and 5 ml amp, 30 ml vial.
2. **Amodiaquine:** For treatment of acute attack of malaria: 25–35 mg/kg over 3 days; CAMOQUIN 200 mg (as HCl = 150 mg base) tab; BASOQUIN 150 mg (base) per 5 ml susp.
3. **Piperaquine:** 960 mg (16 mg/kg) along with dihydroartemisinin 120 mg (2 mg/kg) daily × 3 days (as ACT combination therapy).
4. **Mefloquine:** For treatment of uncomplicated falciparum malaria: 25 mg/kg split into 2 doses taken on 2 days along with 3 days artesunate (4 mg/kg/day) combination therapy; For prophylaxis: 5 mg/kg (max 250 mg) per week started 2 weeks before entering endemic area;
   MEFLOTAS, MEFLIAM, CONFAL, FACITAL 250 mg tab to be taken after meals with plenty of water.
5. **Quinine:** For complicated (Cerebral) malaria: 20 mg/kg diluted in 5% glucose and infused i.v. over 4 hours, followed by 10 mg/kg over 8 hours repeated every 8 hours till patient improves (regains consciousness), followed by oral therapy to complete 7 day course. For uncomplicated falciparum malaria: 600 mg (10 mg/kg) TDS oral for 7 days along with doxycycline 100 mg daily for 7 days or clindamycin 600 mg BD for 7 days;
   REZOQUIN, QUININE; QUINARSOL 300, 600 mg tab, 600 mg/2 ml inj.
6. **Proguanil (chloroguanide):** For malaria prophylaxis: 200 mg daily with chloroquine 300 mg weekly till 4 weeks after exposure; PROGUMAL 100 mg tab.

7. **Pyrimethamine-sulfadoxine:** For treatment of uncomplicated falciparum malaria: 75 mg + 1500 mg single dose; Sulfadoxine 500 mg + pyrimethamine 25 mg tab: LARIDOX, RIMODAR, FANCIDAR, MALOCIDE; REZIZ 500 mg + 25 mg tab and per 10 ml susp (adults 3 tab, children 9–14 yr 2 tab, 4–8 yr 1 tab, 1–4 yr ½ tab); REZIZ FORTE 750 mg + 37.5 mg tab.

   Sulfamethopyrazine 500 mg + **pyrimethamine** 25 mg tab: METAFIN, MALADEX tab.

   Dapsone 100 mg + **pyrimethamine** 25 mg tab; MALOPRIM tab.
8. **Doxycycline:** For treatment of chloroquine resistant falciparum malaria: 100 mg OD combined with quinine or pyrimethamine-sulfadoxine.

   For prophylaxis of chloroquine resistant falciparum malaria in travellers: 100 mg OD (as alternative to mefloquine).
9. **Clindamycin:** 600 mg BD for combination with quinine for chloroquine resistant vivax/falciparum malaria.
10. **Primaquine:** For radical cure of vivax malaria: 15 mg (children 0.25 mg/kg) daily for 2 weeks along with chloroquine for 3 days; As gametocidal for falciparum malaria 45 mg (0.75 mg/kg) single dose along with chloroquine; MALIRID, EVAQUIN (as phosphate 26 mg = 15 mg base) 2.5, 7.5, 15, 45 mg tab.
11. **Artesunate:** oral (for uncomplicated falciparum malaria) 100 mg BD (4 mg/kg/day) × 3 days in combination with mefloquine or sulfadoxine-pyrimethamine as ACT.

    Parenteral (for severe and complicated falciparum malaria) 2.4 mg/kg i.v. or i.m. repeated after 12 and 24 hours and then once daily for 7 days. Switchover to oral ACT in-between whenever patient can take oral medication. FALCIGO, FALCYNATE, ARTINATE 50 mg tab, 60 mg/vial inj., LARINATE, ARNATE 50 mg tab;

    Artesunate 50 mg tab. + **mefloquine** 250 mg tab in kit: FALCIGO PLUS tab kit.

    Artesunate (100 mg) × 6 tab. + **sulfadoxine** (500 mg)-**pyrimethamine** (25 mg) × 3 tab. kit: ZESUNATE kit, MASUNATE kit, FALCIART kit.

    Artesunate 200 mg (4 mg/kg) + **amodiaquine** 600 mg (10 mg/kg) daily × 3 days.

12. **Artemether:** Oral (for uncomplicated falciparum malaria) 80 mg twice daily × 3 days in combination with lumefantrine as ACT (to be taken with fatty meal).

    Parenteral (for severe and complicated falciparum malaria) 3.2 mg/kg i.m. on 1st day, followed by 1.6 mg/kg daily for 7 days. Switch-over to 3 day oral ACT in-between whenever patient can take oral medication; PALUTHER, LARITHER, MALITHER, METHILEX 40 mg cap, 80 mg inj (in 1 ml arachis oil).

    Artemether 20 mg + **lumefantrine** 120 mg tab: COARTEM, LUMETHER, COMBITHER tab, adult and child above 35 kg body weight 4 tab BD, child 25–35 kg 3 tab BD, 15–25 kg 2 tab BD, 5–15 kg 1 tab BD, all for 3 days; Artemether 80 mg + lumefantrine 480 mg tab: FALCIMAX PLUS, ARTE PLUS adults 1 tab BD × 3 days.

13. **Arteether:** (for severe and complicated falciparum malaria) 3.2 mg/kg i.m. on 1st day, followed by 1.6 mg/kg daily for the next 4 days. Switch-over to 3 day oral ACT in-between whenever the patient is able to take oral medication. E-MAL, FALCY, RAPITHER 150 mg/2 ml amp.

14. **Arterolane:** Oral (for uncomplicated falciparum malaria) 150 mg once daily in combination with piperaquine 750 mg once daily × 3 days; SYNRIAM (arterolane 100 mg + piperaquine 750 mg) cap.

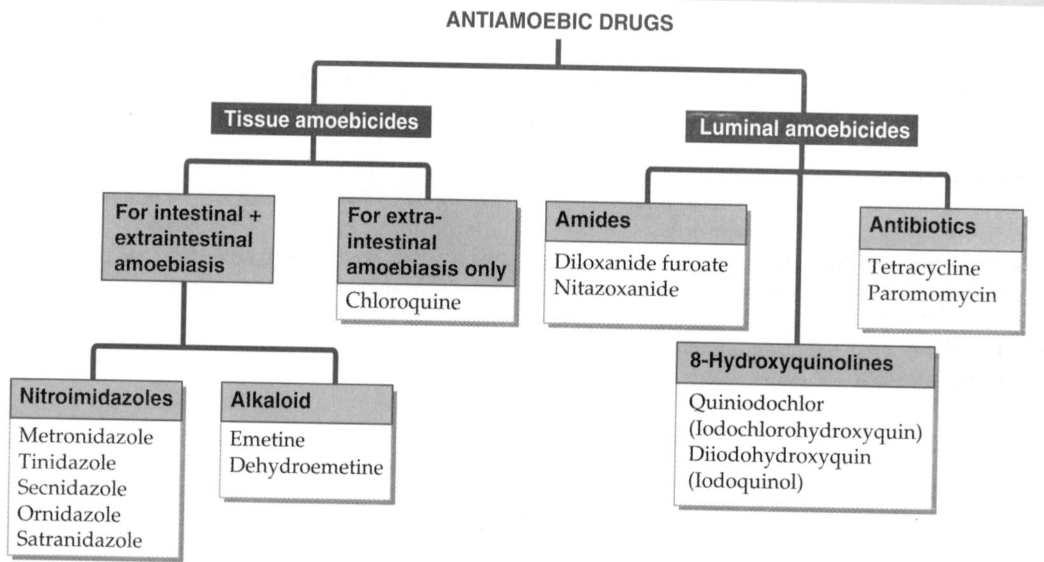
ANTIAMOEBIC DRUGS
Tissue amoebicides
Luminal amoebicides
For intestinal + extraintestinal amoebiasis
For extra-intestinal amoebiasis only
Chloroquine
Amides
Diloxanide furoate
Nitazoxanide
Antibiotics
Tetracycline
Paromomycin
8-Hydroxyquinolines
Quiniodochlor (Iodochlorohydroxyquin)
Diiodohydroxyquin (Iodoquinol)
Nitroimidazoles
Metronidazole
Tinidazole
Secnidazole
Ornidazole
Satranidazole
Alkaloid
Emetine
Dehydroemetine

Preparations

1. **Metronidazole:** *For amoebic dysentery and liver abscess*—800 mg TDS (children 30–50 mg/kg/day) for 7–10 days oral, or 500 mg slow i.v. infusion every 6–8 hours till oral therapy is instituted; *For mild intestinal amoebiasis*—400 mg TDS for 5–7 days. *For serious anaerobic bacterial infections*: 15 mg/kg infused i.v. over 1 hr followed by 7.5 mg/kg every 6 hrs till oral therapy can be instituted with 400–800 mg TDS;
   FLAGYL, METROGYL, METRON, ARISTOGYL, ALDEZOLE 200, 400 mg tab, 200 mg/5 ml susp. (as benzoyl metronidazole: tasteless); 500 mg/100 ml i.v. infusion; UNIMEZOL 200, 400 mg tabs, 200 mg/5 ml susp, METROGYL GEL, LUPIGYL GEL: 1% gel for vaginal/topical application.
2. **Tinidazole:** For *intestinal amoebiasis*: 2 g OD for 3 days (children 30–50 mg/kg/day) or 0.6 g BD for 5–10 days.
   Trichomoniasis and giardiasis: 2 g single dose or 0.6 g OD for 7 days.
   For *Anaerobic infections*:
   prophylactic—2 g single dose before colorectal surgery;
   therapeutic—2 g followed by 0.5 g BD for 5 days oral, 0.8 g i.v. infusion 8–12 hourly.
   For *H. pylori:* 500 mg BD for 1–2 weeks in triple combination;
   TINIBA 300, 500, 1000 mg tabs; 800 mg/400 ml i.v. infusion; TRIDAZOLE 300, 500 mg tab; FASIGYN 0.5 g and 1 g tab, TINI 0.3 g, 0.5 g tabs, 75 mg/5 ml and 150 mg/5 ml oral susp.
3. **Secnidazole:** 2 g single dose (children 30 mg/kg) for intestinal amoebiasis, giardiasis, trichomonas vaginitis and nonspecific bacterial vaginosis; 1.5 g/day for 5 days in acute amoebic dysentery;
   SECNIL, SECZOL 0.5, 1.0 g tabs; NOAMEBA-DS 1.0 g tab.
4. **Ornidazole:** 2 g OD oral for 3 days or 0.6 g BD for 5–10 days; 0.5–1.0 g slow i.v. infusion;
   DAZOLIC 500 mg tab, 500 mg/100 ml vial for i.v. infusion. ORNIDA 500 mg tab, 125 mg/5 ml susp.
5. **Satranidazole:** Amoebiasis: 300 mg BD for 3–5 days, giardiasis and trichomoniasis: 600 mg single dose orally;
   SATROGYL 300 mg tab.

6. **Emetine:** 60 mg i.m./s.c. OD for not more than 10 days; EMETINE HCL 60 mg/2 ml inj.
7. **Dehydroemetine:** 60–100 mg i.m./s.c. OD for not more than 10 days; DEHYDROEMETINE HCL 30 mg/ml inj 1 and 2 ml amps.
8. **Chloroquine:** 600 mg (base) daily for 2 days followed by 300 mg OD for 2–3 weeks.
9. **Diloxanide furoate:** 500 mg TDS for 5–10 days; children 20 mg/kg/day;
   FURAMIDE, AMICLINE 0.5 g tab; in TINIBA–DF 250 mg + 150 mg tinidazole and TINIBA-DF FORTE 500 mg + 300 mg tabs; in ENTAMIZOLE 250 mg + 200 mg metronidazole and ENTAMIZOLE FORTE 500 mg + 400 mg tabs.
10. **Nitazoxanide:** 500 mg (children 7.5 mg/kg) BD × 3 days.
    NITACURE, NITCOL, NITARID 200, 500 mg tabs, 100 mg/5 ml dry syrup.
11. **Quiniodochlor (Iodochlorohydroxyquin, Clioquinol):** 250–500 mg TDS;
    ENTEROQUINOL, QUINOFORM 250 mg tab.
12. **Diiodohydroxyquin (Iodoquinol):** 650 mg TDS; not to exceed 2.0 g per day for 14 days; DIODOQUIN 650 mg tab, 210 mg/5 ml susp.
13. **Tetracycline/Oxytetracycline:** 250 mg QID oral.

Drugs for Giardiasis

1. **Metronidazole:** 400 mg TDS (children 15 mg/kg/day) for 5–7 days or 2 g daily for 3 days.
2. **Tinidazole/Secnidazole:** 2 g single dose or 0.6 g daily for 7 days.
3. **Nitazoxanide:** 500 mg (children 7.5 mg/kg) BD × 3 days.
4. **Quiniodochlor:** 250 mg TDS for 7 days.
5. **Furazolidone:** 100 mg TDS for 5–7 days; FUROXONE 100 mg tab, 25 mg/5 ml susp.

Drugs for Trichomoniasis

A. Drugs used orally

1. Metronidazole: 400 mg TDS for 7 days or 2 g single dose.
2. Tinidazole: 600 mg OD for 7 days or 2 g single dose.
3. Secnidazole: 2 g single dose.

B. Drugs used intravaginally

1. **Diiodohydroxyquin:** 200 mg inserted intravaginally at bed time for 1–2 weeks; FLORAQUIN 100 mg vaginal pessaries.
2. **Quiniodochlor:** 200 mg inserted in the vagina every night for 1–3 weeks; GYNOSAN 200 mg vaginal tab.
3. **Metronidazole:** 1% topical gel applied in vagina once or twice daily; METROGYL GEL, LUPIGYL GEL 1%.
4. **Povidone-iodine:** 400 mg inserted in the vagina daily at night for 2 weeks; BETADINE VAGINAL 200 mg pessaries.

Drugs for Leishmaniasis (Kala azar)

1. **Amphotericin B deoxycholate:** 0.75–1.0 mg/kg i.v. infusion over 4 hours daily/on alternate days till 15 mg/kg total dose.
2. **Liposomal amphotericin B:** 3–5 mg/kg i.v. infusion daily for 3–5 days (total dose 15 mg/kg)
3. **Miltefosine:** 50 mg cap twice daily orally; children (2–11 years) 2.5 mg/kg/day.
4. **Paromomycin sulfate:** 15 mg/kg i.m. OD for 21 days.
5. **Sodium stibogluconate:** 20 mg/kg i.m. or slow i.v. daily for 30 days (in areas with *Leishmania* sensitive to stibogluconate).

Combinations

1. Liposomal amphotericin B (5 mg/kg i.v. infusion single dose) + Miltefosine (100 mg/day oral for 7 days)
2. Liposomal amphotericin B (5 mg/kg i.v. infusion single dose) + Paromomycin (15 mg/kg i.m. daily for 10 days)
3. Miltefosine (100 mg/day oral for 10 days) + Paromomycin (15 mg/kg i.m. daily for 10 days).

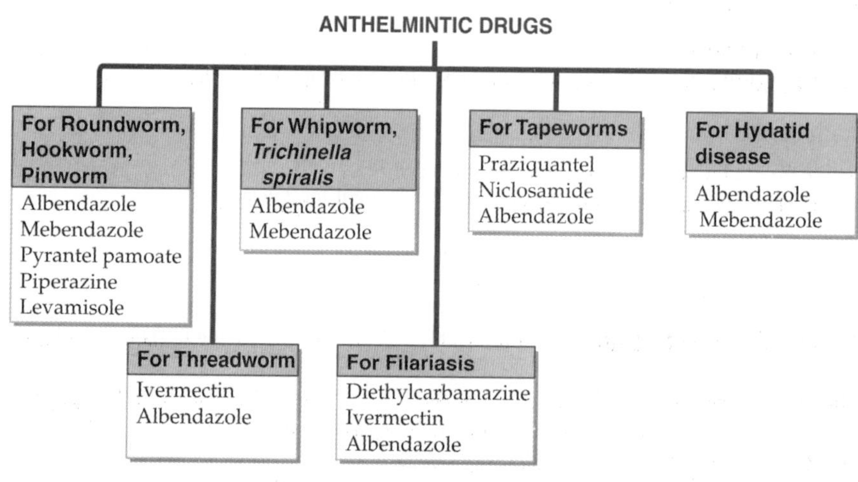

Preparations

1. Mebendazole: For round worm, hookworm and whipworm (*Trichuris*) 100 mg BD for 3 days; for pinworm 100 mg single dose repeated after 2–3 weeks; for *Trichinella spiralis* 200 mg BD for 4 days; for hydatid disease 200–400 mg BD–TDS for 3–4 weeks; children 1–2 year age 1/2 dose;
   MEBEX, WORMIN 100 mg chewale tab, 100 mg/5 ml susp, MEBAZOLE 100 mg tab.
2. Albendazole: For roundworm, hookworm, pinworm and whipworm 400 mg single dose (for children 1–2 years 1/2 dose); for tapeworms, strongyloidosis and trichinosis 400 mg daily for 3 days; neurocysticercosis 15 mg/kg daily for 8–15 days (with corticosteroids); hydatid disease 400 mg BD for 4 weeks (upto 3 courses with 2 weeks gap); ZENTEL, ALMINTH, ALBEZOLE 400 mg tab, 200 mg/5 ml susp.
3. Pyrantel pamoate: For roundworm, *Ancylostoma* and pinworm 10 mg/kg single dose, for *Necator* and strongyloidosis 10 mg/kg daily for 3 days; NEMOCID, ANTIMINTH, EXPENT 250 mg tab, 500 mg/10 ml susp.
4. Piperazine: For roundworm infestation 4 g once a day for 2 consecutive days; children 0.75 g/year of age (max. 4 g). Enterobiasis—50 mg/kg (max. 2 g) once a day for 7 days or 75 mg/kg (max. 4 g) single dose, repeated after 3 weeks.
   PIPERAZINE CITRATE; 0.75 g/5 ml elixir in 30 ml, 115 ml bottle; 0.5 g (as phosphate) tablets.
5. Levamisole: For roundworm 150 mg (adults), 100 mg (children 20–39 kg body weight), 50 mg (children 10–19 kg weight) single dose, for *Ancylostoma* 2 doses 12 hour apart;
   DEWORMIS, VERMISOL 50, 150 mg tabs, 50 mg/5 ml syr.
6. Diethylcarbamazine citrate: For filariasis 2 mg/kg TDS for 12–21 days, for tropical eosinophilia 2–4 mg/kg TDS for 2–3 weeks; HETRAZAN, BANOCIDE 50, 100 mg tabs, 120 mg/5 ml syr, 50 mg/5 ml pediatric syr.
7. Ivermectin: 10–15 mg (0.15–0.2 mg/kg) orally single dose for strongyloidosis, enterobiasis, ascariasis as well as scabies and pediculosis; for filariasis and onchocerciasis 0.2 mg/kg is repeated annually along with albendazole 400 mg; IVERMECTOL, IVERMEC, VERMIN 3, 6 mg tabs, to be taken on empty stomach.

8. **Niclosamide:** For tapeworm (*T. solium, T. saginata*) 2.0 g taken in 2 doses 1 hour apart (children 2–6 years 1.0 g total dose) followed by a saline purge after 2 hours; for *H. nana* 2.0 g repeated daily for 5 days;
NICLOSAN 0.5 g tab (to be chewed and swallowed with water).
9. **Praziquantel:** For tapeworm (*T. solium, T. saginata*) 10 mg/kg single dose in the morning; for *H. nana* and *D. latum* 15–25 mg/kg single dose in the morning; for neurocysticercosis 50 mg/kg/day in 3 divided doses for 15 days; for Schistosomiasis 40–75 mg/kg in one day; for other flukes 75 mg/kg in one day for 1–2 days;
CYSTICIDE 500 mg tab, DISTOCIDE 600 mg tab.

13 Anticancer Drugs (Antineoplastic Drugs)

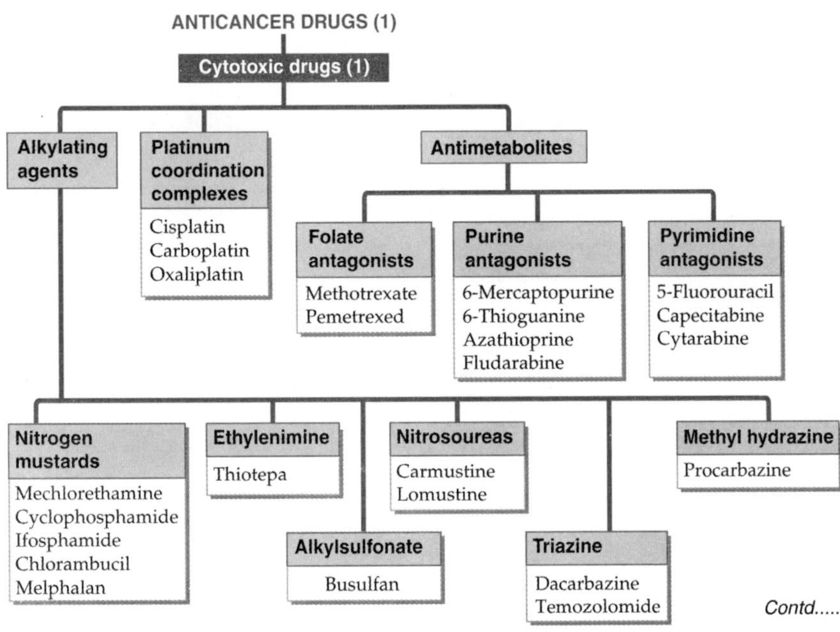

Contd.....

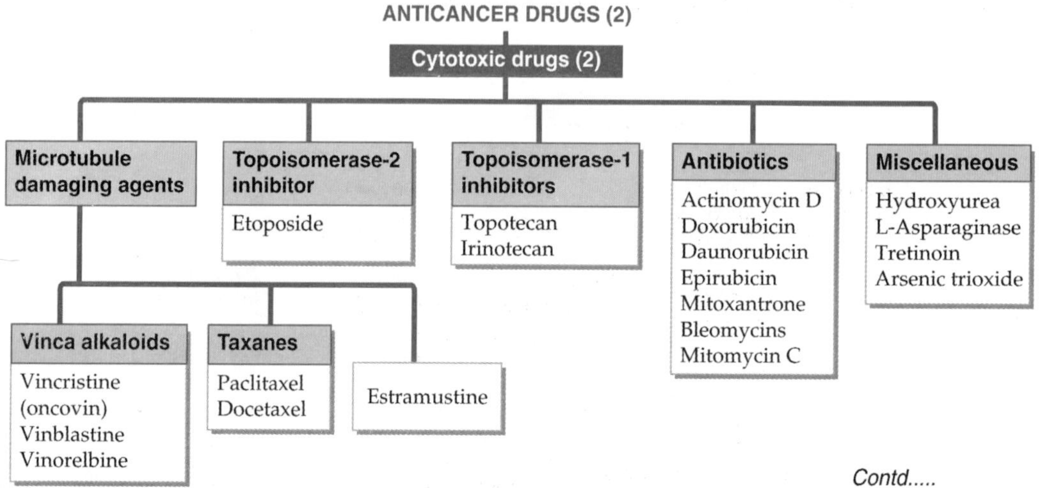
ANTICANCER DRUGS (2)
Cytotoxic drugs (2)
Microtubule damaging agents
Topoisomerase-2 inhibitor
Etoposide
Topoisomerase-1 inhibitors
Topotecan
Irinotecan
Antibiotics
Actinomycin D
Doxorubicin
Daunorubicin
Epirubicin
Mitoxantrone
Bleomycins
Mitomycin C
Miscellaneous
Hydroxyurea
L-Asparaginase
Tretinoin
Arsenic trioxide
Vinca alkaloids
Vincristine (oncovin)
Vinblastine
Vinorelbine
Taxanes
Paclitaxel
Docetaxel
Estramustine

Contd.....

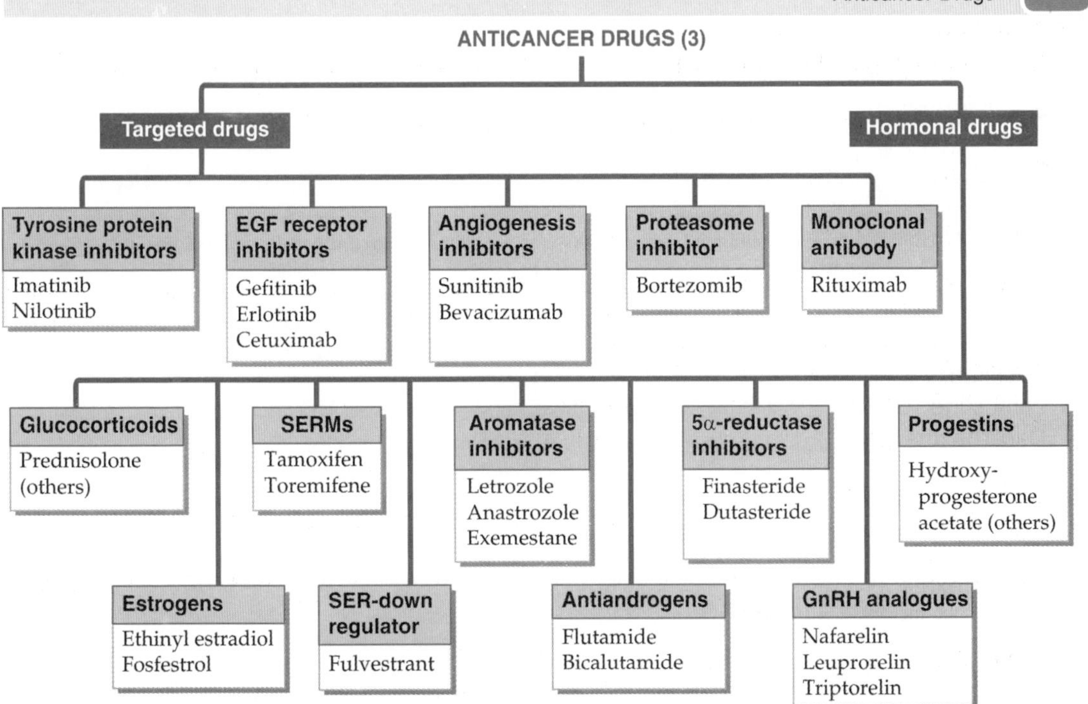
ANTICANCER DRUGS (3)
Targeted drugs
Hormonal drugs
Tyrosine protein kinase inhibitors
Imatinib
Nilotinib
EGF receptor inhibitors
Gefitinib
Erlotinib
Cetuximab
Angiogenesis inhibitors
Sunitinib
Bevacizumab
Proteasome inhibitor
Bortezomib
Monoclonal antibody
Rituximab
Glucocorticoids
Prednisolone (others)
SERMs
Tamoxifen
Toremifene
Aromatase inhibitors
Letrozole
Anastrozole
Exemestane
5α-reductase inhibitors
Finasteride
Dutasteride
Progestins
Hydroxy-progesterone acetate (others)
Estrogens
Ethinyl estradiol
Fosfestrol
SER-down regulator
Fulvestrant
Antiandrogens
Flutamide
Bicalutamide
GnRH analogues
Nafarelin
Leuprorelin
Triptorelin

Preparations

1. **Mechlorethamine (Mustine HCl):** 0.1 mg/kg i.v. daily × 4 days; courses may be repeated at suitable intervals; MUSTINE 10 mg dry powder in vial.
2. **Cyclophosphamide:** 2–3 mg/kg/day oral; 10–15 mg/kg i.v. every 7–10 days, i.m. use also possible; ENDOXAN, CYCLOXAN 50 mg tab; 200, 500, 1000 mg inj.
3. **Ifosfamide:** 10–15 mg/kg i.v.; HOLOXAN, IPAMIDE 1 g vial, HOLOXAN-UROMITEXAN 1 g vial + 3 amps of mesna 200 mg inj.
4. **Chlorambucil:** 4–10 mg (0.1–0.2 mg/kg) oral daily for 3–6 weeks, then 2 mg daily for maintenance; LEUKERAN 2, 5 mg tab.
5. **Melphalan:** 10 mg daily for 7 days or 6 mg/day for 2–3 weeks—4 weeks gap—2 to 4 mg daily for maintenance orally. Also used for regional perfusion in malignant melanoma; ALKERAN 2, 5 mg tab, 50 mg per vial for inj.
6. **Thio-TEPA:** 0.3–0.4 mg/kg i.v. at 1–4 week intervals; THIOTEPA 15 mg per vial inj.
7. **Busulfan:** 2–6 mg/day (0.06 mg/kg/day) orally; MYLERAN, BUSUPHAN 2 mg tab.
8. **Lomustine (CCNU):** 100–130 mg/m^2 BSA single oral dose every 6 weeks; LOMUSTINE 40, 100 mg cap.
9. **Dacarbazine (DTIC):** 3.5 mg/kg/day i.v. for 10 days, repeat after 4 weeks; DACARIN 100, 200, 500 mg inj; DACARZINE 200 mg/vial inj.
10. **Temozolamide:** 100–250 mg/day; GLIOZ 20, 100, 250 mg caps.
11. **Procarbazine:** 100 mg/m$^{2/}$day for 14 days in 28 day cycles; INDICARB 20 mg cap, NEOZINE, P-CARZINE 50 mg cap.
12. **Methotrexate:** 15–30 mg/day for 5 days orally or 20–40 mg/m^2 body surface area (BSA) i.m./i.v. twice weekly, maintenance therapy 2.5–15 mg/day; NEOTREXATE 2.5 mg tab, 50 mg/2 ml inj; BIOTREXATE 2.5 mg tab, 5, 15, 50 mg/vial inj.
13. **Pemetrexed:** 500 mg/m^2 i.v. every 3 weeks; PEMEX 500 mg vial for i.v. inj.

14. **6-Mercaptopurine:** 2.5 mg/kg/day orally, half dose for maintenance;
PURINETHOL, EMPURINE, 6-MP 50 mg tab.
15. **6-Thioguanine:** 100–200 mg/m^2/day oral for 5–20 days; 6–TG 40 mg tab.
16. **Azathioprine:** 3–5 mg/kg/day oral, maintenance 1–2 mg/kg/day;
IMURAN, TRANSIMUNE, AZOPRINE 50 mg tab.
17. **Fludarabine:** 25 mg/m^2 BSA daily for 5 days every 28 days by i.v. infusion, FLUDARA 50 mg/vial inj.
18. **Fluorouracil (5-FU):** 500 mg/m^2 i.v. infusion over 1–3 hours weekly for 6–8 weeks, or 12 mg/kg/day i.v. for 4 days followed by 6 mg/kg i.v. on alternate days 3–4 doses;
FLURACIL, FIVE FLURO, FIVOCIL 250 mg/5 ml and 500 mg/10 ml vial for i.v. inj.
19. **Cytarabine:** 100 mg/m^2 i.v. injection OD/BD for 5–10 days, or 1–3 g/day;
REMCYTA, CYTROSAR, CYTABIN 100, 500, 1000 mg inj.
20. **Vincristine (Oncovin):** 1.5–2 mg/m^2 BSA i.v. weekly; ONCOCRISTIN, CYTOCRISTIN 1 mg/vial inj.
21. **Vinblastine:** 0.1–0.15 mg/kg i.v. weekly × 3 doses; UNIBLASTIN, CYTOBLASTIN 10 mg/vial inj.
22. **Vinorelbine:** 25–30 mg/m^2 weekly by slow i.v. inj over 10 min; VINOTEC, RELBOVIN 10 mg, 50 mg vial.
23. **Paclitaxel:** 135–175 mg/m^2 by i.v. infusion over 3 hr, repeated every 3 weeks; ALTAXEL, MITOTAX, ONCOTAXEL 30, 100, 260 mg as 6 mg/ml in cremophor emulsion (polyoxyethylated castor oil + alcohol + water).
24. **Docetaxel:** 75–100 mg/m^2 i.v. over 1 hr; repeat at 3 weeks;
DOCECAD, DOCETERE, DOXEL 20, 80, 120 mg/vial inj.
25. **Etoposide:** 50–100 mg/m^2/day i.v. for 5 days, 100–200 mg/day oral; PELTASOL 100 mg in 5 ml inj., LASTET 25, 50, 100 mg cap, 100 mg/5 ml inj, ACTITOP 50, 100 mg caps, 100 mg/5 ml inj.
26. **Estramustine:** 4–5 mg/kg oral TDS; ESMUST, ESTRAM 140 mg cap.
27. **Topotecan:** 1.5 mg/m^2 i.v. over 30 min daily for 5 days; TOPOTEC, CANTOP 2.5 mg inj.

28. **Irinotecan:** 125 mg/m^2 i.v. over 90 min weekly for 4 weeks;
IRINOTEL, IRNOCAM 40 mg (2 ml), 100 mg (5 ml) inj.
29. **Actinomycin D (Dactinomycin):** 15 μg/kg i.v. daily for 5 days; DACMOZEN 0.5 mg/vial inj.
30. **Daunorubicin (Rubidomycin):** 30–50 mg/m^2 BSA i.v. daily for 3 days, repeat after 3–4 weeks.
DAUNOCIN, DAUNOMYCIN 20 mg/vial inj.
31. **Doxorubicin:** 60–75 mg/m^2 BSA slow i.v. injection every 3 weeks;
ADRIAMYCIN, DOXORUBICIN, ONCODRIA 10 mg, 50 mg per vial inj.
32. **Epirubicin:** 60–90 mg/m^2 i.v. over 5 min, repeated at 3 weeks; total dose <900 mg/m^2.
ALRUBICIN, EPIRUBITEC 10, 50 mg vials for reconstitution with diluent.
33. **Mitoxantrone:** 14 mg/m^2 single i.v. dose, repeat at 3 weeks; ONCOTRON 20 mg/10 ml inj.
34. **Bleomycin:** 30 mg twice weekly i.v. or i.m. (total dose 300–400 mg); BLEOCIN, ONCOBLEO 15 mg inj.
35. **Mitomycin C:** 10 mg/m^2 BSA, infused i.v. in one day or divided in 5 and infused over 5 days;
MITOCIN, ALMITO, LYOMIT 2, 10 mg inj.
36. **Hydroxyurea:** 20–30 mg/kg daily or 80 mg/kg twice weekly oral;
CYTODROX, HONDREA, UNIDREA 500 mg cap.
37. **L-Asparaginase:** 50–200 KU/kg i.v. or i.m. daily for 3–4 weeks; LEUNASE, HOILASP 10,000 KU per vial inj.
38. **Cisplatin:** 50–100 mg/m^2 BSA by slow i.v. infusion every 3–4 weeks;
CISPLATIN, CISPLAT, PLATINEX 10 mg/10 ml, 50 mg/50 ml vial.
39. **Carboplatin:** 400 mg/m^2 as an i.v. infusion over 15–60 min, to be repeated only after 4 weeks;
ONCOCARBIN, KEMOCARB 150, 450 mg/vial inj.

40. **Oxaliplatin:** 85 mg/m^2 i.v. every 2 weeks; KINAPLAT, OPLATIN 50 mg in 25 ml and 100 mg in 50 ml vial.
41. **Imatinib:** 400 mg/day with meal; for accelerated phase of CML 600-800 mg/day; IMATIB-α, SHANTINIB, GLEE-VEC, UNITINIB 100, 400 mg caps.
42. **Gefitinib:** 250 mg/day oral; GEFONIB, GEFTINAT 250 mg tab/cap.
43. **Erlotinib:** 100–150 mg OD 1 hour before or 2 hours after meal; ERLOTEC 100, 150 mg tabs.
44. **Bortezomib:** 1.3 mg/m^2 i.v. bolus injection, 4 doses at 3 day intervals; EGYBORT 3.5 mg/vial inj.

Note: *See* Index for preparations of hormones and hormone antagonists

14 Miscellaneous Drugs

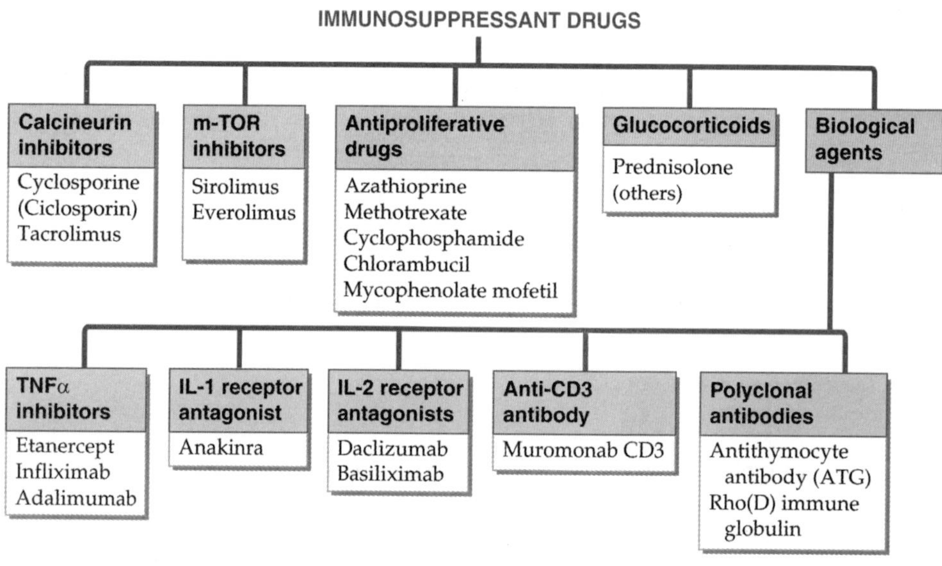

Preparations

1. **Cyclosporine:** 10–15 mg/kg/day with milk or fruit juice till 1–2 weeks after transplantation, gradually reduced to maintenance dose of 2–6 mg/kg/day. Therapy may be started with 3–5 mg/kg i.v. infusion.
   IMUSPORIN 25, 50, 100 mg soft gelatin cap; microemulsion formulation SANDIMMUN NEORAL, PANIMUN BIORAL 25, 50, 100 mg caps; SANDIMMUN, PANIMUN 100 mg/ml inj in 1 ml, 5 ml, 50 ml vials dispersed in cremaphor emulsion to be diluted and infused i.v. over 4–6 hours.
2. **Tacrolimus:** 0.05–0.1 mg/kg 12 hourly oral (for renal transplantation) 0.1-0.2 mg/kg (for liver transplantation);
   PANGRAF, TACROMUS 0.5, 1.0, 5.0 mg caps; TACRODERM, TACREL 0.03, 0.1% oint.
3. **Sirolimus:** Loading dose 1 mg/m^2 orally daily, followed by titrated lower doses for maintenance; RAPACAN 1 mg tab.
4. **Azathioprine:** Initially 3–5 mg/kg/day oral, followed by 1–2 mg/kg/day for maintenance.
5. **Cyclophosphamide:** 10–15 mg/kg i.v., 2–3 mg/kg/day oral.
6. **Methotrexate:** Initially 15–30 mg/day oral, 2.5–15 mg/day for maintenance.
7. **Chlorambucil:** 2–10 mg/day oral.
8. **Mycophenolate mofetil:** 1 g oral twice daily; CELLMUNE, MYCEPT, MYCOFIT 250, 500 mg tab/cap.
9. **Etanercept:** 25–50 mg s.c. once or twice weekly; ENBREL, ENBROL 25 mg in 0.5 ml and 50 mg in 1 ml inj.
10. **Antithymocyte globulin:** LYMPHOGLOBULIN (equine) 100 mg/vial inj.; 10 mg/kg/day i.v.;
    THYMOGLOBULIN (rabbit) 25 mg/vial inj.; 1.5 mg/kg/day; ATG 100 mg inj; 200 mg i.v./day.
11. **Rho(D) immune globulin:** 250–350 µg i.m. of freez dried preparation.
    RHIGGAL 100, 350 µg vial, RHESUMAN, RHOGAM, IMOGAM 300 µg per vial and prefilled syringe.

Note: *See* Index for preparations of other drugs.

CHELATING AGENTS

1. Dimercaprol (British Antilewisite, BAL): 5 mg/kg, followed by 2–3 mg/kg every 4–8 hours for 2 days and then once daily for 10 days injected i.m.; BAL INJ 100 mg/2 ml in arachis oil inj.
2. Dimercaptosuccinic acid (Succimer).
3. Calcium disodium edetate (Ca Na_2 EDTA): 1 g diluted in 200–300 ml saline and infused i.v. over 1 hour twice daily for 3–5 days, to be repeated after a week.
4. Calcium disodium DTPA.
5. Penicillamine: 0.5–1 g daily in divided doses 1 hour before or 2 hour after meals to avoid chelation of dietary metals; ARTAMIN, CILAMIN 250 mg cap, ARTIN 150, 250 mg cap.
6. Desferrioxamine: For acute iron poisoning: 0.5–1 g (50 mg/kg) i.m. 4–12 hourly as required or 10–15 mg/kg/hour (max 75 mg/kg in one day) i.v. infusion; for transfusion siderosis in thalassemia patients 0.5–1 g/day i.m.; DESFERAL 0.5 g/vial inj.
7. Deferiprone: 50–100 mg/kg oral daily in 2–4 divided doses; KELFER 250, 500 mg caps.

LOCALLY ACTING DRUGS ON SKIN AND MUCOUS MEMBRANES

A. Demulcents

1. Gum Acacia: as 2–4% pseudosolution in water.
2. Gum Tragacanth: as 2–4% pseudosolution in water.
3. Glycyrrhiza: as glycyrrhiza dry extract 1–2 g or liquid extract 2–4 ml, in lozenges and mixtures.
4. Methylcellulose: 0.5% in nose drops and contact lens solution; CADILOSE 0.5% drops in 10 ml bottle.

5. Propylene glycol: 50% in water.
6. Glycerine: 10–50% in water.

B. Emollients

1. *Vegetable oils*: Olive oil, Arachis oil, Sesame oil, Cocoa butter
2. *Animal products:* Wool fat, Lard, Bees wax, Spermaceti
3. *Petroleum products:* Paraffin wax (soft/hard), Liquid paraffin.

C. Adsorbants and Protectives

1. *Dermal protectives:* Magnesium stearate, Zinc stearate, Talc, Calamine, Zinc oxide, Bentonite, Starch, Boric acid, Aloe-vera gel.
2. *Occlusive protectives:* Polyvinyl polymer, Feracrylum, Dimethicone, Sucralfate.

Preparations

CALADRYL: Calamine 8% diphenhydramine 1%, Camphor 0.1% lotion.
CALAK, CALMIS (Calamine lotion): Calamine 15%, zinc oxide 5%, bentonite 3%, sodium citrate 0.5%, liquified phenol 0.5%, glycerin 5% lotion.
CALACREME 5% cream, CALAMINOL: 5% emulsion.
ALOVIT: Aloe extract 10%, Vit E 0.5% cream.
ALOEDERM: Aloe juice 10%, vit E acetate 0.2%, sesame oil 2% cream.
JULA: Aloe vera juice gel 50% gel.
LUBRIDERM-SF: Dimethicone 4%, vit E acetate 1%, vegetable oil 2%, propylene glycol 10% cream.
HEALEX SPRAY: Polyvinyl polymer 2.5% + benzocaine 0.36% as aerosol wound dressing.

SEPGARD GEL: Feracrylum 1% gel, to be applied as a thin film on the abrasion/wound.
SILENT-SF: White soft paraffin 2.5%, dimethicone 0.5% cream.
BARRIER-SF: Dimethicone 15%, vita E acetate 0.18% cream.
PEPSIGARD LIGHT GEL: Sucralfate 10% gel.

D. Astringents

1. *Vegetable astringents*
   Tannic acid: as glycerine of tannic acid 25%
   Tannins: as tincture catechu, tea leaf infusion
2. *Alcohols*
   Ethanol, Methanol, Propanol
3. *Mineral astringents*
   Alum, Aluminium hydroxychloride, Zinc oxide, Zirconyl hydroxychloride

E. Counterirritants

1. *Volatile oils*
   Turpentine oil, Eucalyptus oil, Clove oil
2. *Stearoptenes*
   Camphor, Thymol, Menthol
3. *Other counterirritants*
   Mustard seeds (as mustard plaster), Capsicum, Canthridin, Methylsalicylate, Alcohol

Preparations

ALGIPAN: Capsicum oleoresin 0.1%, histamine 0.1%, methyl nicotinate 1%, glycol salicylate 5% cream.
RELISPRAY: Wintergreen oil (methyl salicylate) 20%, clove oil 1%, Menthol 4%, Nilgiri oil 6%, Camphor 10%, Cinnamon oil 0.5%, terpentine oil 10% spray
ARJET SPRAY: Methyl salicylate 875 mg, menthol 1.6 g, camphor 1.5 g, benzyl nicotinate 20 mg, squalance 250 mg, glycol salicylate 875 mg per 50 ml spray.
EUTHERIA: Eucalyptol 7.2%, menthol 4.7%, methylsalicylate 11.25% balm.
MEDICREME: Methylsalicylate 8%, menthol 2%, adrenaline 0.03%, mephenesin 2.5%, chlorpheniramine 0.2%, cream.
RELAXYL: Capsicum oleoresin 0.05%, mephenesin 10%, methyl nicotinate 1% ointment.
VICKS VAPORUB: Menthol 2.8%, camphor 5.25%, thymol 0.1% turpentine oil 5.5% ointment.
IODEX: Methylsalicylate 5%, iodine 4% nonstaining ointment.
AMRUTANJAN: Eucalyptus oil 17%, camphor 10%, thymol 1%, menthol 4.5%, methylsalicylate 7% ointment.
CAPSIGYL-D: Capsaicin 0.075%, methyl salicylate 20%, menthol 10%, camphor 5%, eucalyptus oil 5%, diclofenac 1% gel.

F. Keratolytics and Caustics

Salicylic acid, Resorcinol, Podophyllum resin, Silver nitrate, Phenol, Trichloracetic acid, Glacial acetic acid.

Preparations

CORNAC: Salicylic acid 16.5% liquid.
CORN CAP: Salicylic acid 40% ointment in adhesive tape.
FOOT POWDER: Salicylic acid 2% dusting powder.
WHITFIELD-SF: Salicylic acid 3% benzoic acid 6% oint.
PODOWART: Podophyllum renin 20% paint.
CONDYLINE: Podophyllotoxin 0.5% solution.

G. Antiseborrheics

Selenium sulfide, Zinc pyrithione, Sulfur, Resorcinol, Coal tar, Ketoconazole, Clotrimazole, Topical corticosteroids.

Preparations

SELSUN: Slenium sulfide 2.5% susp.
SELDRUFF PLUS: Selenium sulfide 2.5%, clotrimazole 1% susp.
SCALPE: Zinc pyrithione 1%, ketoconazole 2% shampoo.
KETOVATE, NIZRAL: Ketoconazole 2% cream, 2% shampoo.
CANDID-TV SUSP: Selenium disulfide 2.5%, clotrimazole 1% susp.

H. Melanizing agents

1. Psoralen: 10–20 mg (0.3–0.6 mg/kg) orally followed 2 hours later by 15–30 min of exposure to sunlight/UV light; 0.25–1% local application on vitiliginous lesion followed by 1 min (initially) exposure to sunlight; exposure time is increased gradually as tolerated; MANADERM 10 mg tab, 1% oint, PSORLINE 5 mg tab, 0.25% solution, 0.25% oint.
2. Methoxsalen: MACSORALEN 10 mg tab, 1% solution, MELANOCYL 10 mg tab, 0.75% solution, 0.75% with paraminobenzoic acid 2% oint. Use similar to psoralen.
3. Trioxsalen: NEOSORALEN 5, 25 mg tabs, 0.2% lotion. Use similar to psoralen.

I. Demelanizing agents

1. Hydroquinone: 2–6% topical application; EUKROMA 4% cream, MELALITE: Hydroquinone 2% with glyceryl-ester of PABA 2.8% cream, BRITE: hydroquinone 4%, glyceryl PABA 2.8% cream.
2. Monobenzone: 5–20% topical application; BENOQUIN 20% oint.
3. Azelaic acid: 10–20% topical application; AZIDERM 10%, 20% cream.

J. Sunscreens

1. *Chemical sunscreens*

   Para-aminobenzoic acid (PABA): 5–10% topical application; PABALAK 5% solution, PARAMINOL 10% cream.

   Oxybenzone: 2–6% topical application.

   Octyl methoxy cinnamate: 5% topical application;

   EUKROMA-SG: Oxybenzone 3%, Octyl methoxycinnamate 5%, hydroquinone 2% cream.

   SUNSHIELD: Octyl methoxycinnamae 5% , Vit E 0.25% lotion.

2. *Physical sunscreens*

   Petroleum jelly (heavy), Titanium dioxide, Zinc oxide, Calamine

   MELASCREEN: Titanium dioxide, Zinc oxide, Octyl methoxy-cinnamate, benzophenone, avobenzone lotion/cream.

K. Drugs for Psoriasis

1. Topical corticosteroids: (*See* p. 44, 46)
2. Calcipotriol: 0.005% topical application on the lesions only; DAIVONEX 0.005% oint.
3. Tazarotene: 0.05-0.1% topical application daily in the evening;
   LATEZ 0.05% gel, 0.1% cream, TAZRET 0.05%, 0.1% cream.
4. Coaltar: 1–6% topical application;
   EXTAR: Coaltar 6%, Salicylic acid 3%, Sulfur ppt 3% oint; TARSYL: Coaltar 1%, Salicylic acid 3% lotion, IONAX-T coaltar 4.25%, salicylic acid 2% scalp lotion.
5. Acitretin: 0.5-0.75 mg/kg/day oral; ACITRIN, ACETEC, ACERET 10, 25 mg tabs.
6. Psoralen-ultraviolet A (PUVA) therapy
7. *Immunosuppressants:* Methotrexate, Etanercept.

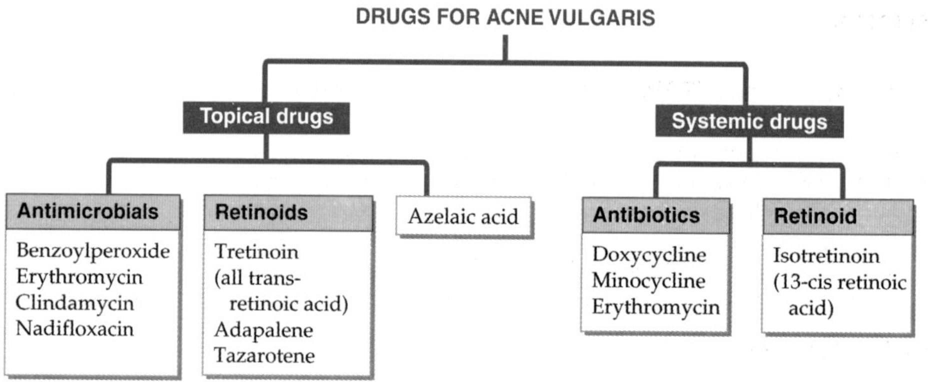

Preparations

1. **Benzoyl peroxide:** 2.5–10% topical application; PERSOL, PERNOX, BENZAC-AC 2.5% and 5% gel; in PERSOL FORTE 10% cream with sulfur ppt. 5%.
2. **Tretinoin (Retinoic acid, all trans vitamin A acid):** 0.025%–0.05% topical application; EUDYNA 0.05% cream, RETINO-A 0.025% and 0.05% cream.
3. **Adapalene:** 0.1% topical application once daily at bed time; ADAFERIN, ADAPEN, ACLENE 0.1% gel.
4. **Azelaic acid:** 10–20% topical application; AZIDERM 10%, 20% cream.
5. **Erythromycin:** 2–4% topical application; ACNEDERM 2% lotion and oint; ERYTOP 3% lotion and cream; EROMED 2% lotion, 4% gel, ACNELAC-Z 4% lotion and gel with zinc acetate 2%.

6. **Clindamycin:** 1% topical application; CLINDAC-A, ACNESOL 1% gel and solution.
7. **Nadifloxacin:** 1% topical application; NADIBACT, NADOXIN 1% topical cream
8. **Isotretinoin (13-cis retinoic acid)** 0.5–1 mg/kg/day; ISOTRETIN, SOTRET 10, 20 mg cap, IRET 20 mg cap.

ANTISEPTICS AND DISINFECTANTS

1. *Phenol derivatives*:
   Phenol, Cresol, Hexylresorcinol, Chloroxylenol, Hexachlorophene.
2. *Oxidizing agents*:
   Pot. permangnate, Hydrogen peroxide, Benzoyl peroxide.
3. *Halogens*:
   Iodine, Iodophores, Chlorine, Chlorophores.
4. *Biguanide*
   Chlorhexidine.
5. *Quaternary ammonium (Cationic);*
   Cetrimide, Benzalkonium chloride (Zephiran), Dequalinium chloride.
6. *Soaps*
   of Sod. and Pot.
7. *Alcohols*
   Ethanol, Isopropanol.
8. *Aldehydes*
   Formaldehyde, Glutaraldehyde.

9. *Acids*

   Boric acid, Acetic acid.
10. *Metallic salts*

    Silver nitrate, Silver sulfadiazine, Mild silver protein, Zinc sulfate, Calamine, Zinc oxide.
11. *Dyes*

    Gentian violet, Brilliant green, Acriflavine, Proflavine.
12. *Furan derivative*

    Nitrofurazone.

Preparations

1. Phenol: 1–5%
2. Cresol: 0.5–4%; LYSOL 50% emulsion of cresol.
3. Chloroxylenol: 0.5–5%; DETTOL 4.8% solution, 0.8% cream, 0.8% soap, 1.4% lubricating obstetric cream, DETTOLIN 1% mouthwash
4. Hexachlorophene: 0.2–3.0% in soaps, dusting powder, etc.
5. Potassium permangnate: as 1:4000–1:10,000 aqueous solution (Condy's lotion).
6. Hydrogen peroxide: 10–30%
7. Iodine: 2% as Tincture iodine (alcoholic solution), 1.25% in Mandel's throat paint; IODEX 4% nonstaining oint.
8. Povidone iodine: 1–10%;

   BETADINE 5% solution, 5% ointment, 5% cream, 7.5% scrub solution, 5% powder, 10% paint, 2% gargle, 200 mg vaginal pessary; PIODIN 10% solution, 10% cream, 1% mouth wash; RANVIDONE AEROSOL 5% spray with freon propellant.

9. **Chlorine:** 0.2–0.4 parts per million (ppm).
10. **Chlorinated lime:** BLEACHING POWDER (30% chlorine).
11. **Sodium hypochlorite:** 4–6% solution.
12. **Chlorhexidine:** 0.1–1.5% solution; CHLODIN, HEXIL, REXIDIN, FLUDENT-CH 0.2% mouth wash.
13. **Cetrimide:** 0.5–3% solution.
    CETAVLON CONCENTRATE: Cetrimide 20%
    SAVLON LIQUID ANTISEPTIC: Chlorhexidine gluconate 1.5% + Cetrimide 3%.
    SAVLON/CETAVLEX CREAM: Chlorhexidine HCl 0.1% + Cetrimide 0.5%.
    SAVLON HOSPITAL CONCENTRATE: Chlorhexidine gluconate 7.5% + Cetrimide 15%.
14. **Dequalinium chloride:** 0.25–1.0%; DEQUADIN 0.25 mg lozenges.
15. **Ethanol:** 70–90%
16. **Isopropanol:** 70–90%
17. **Formaldehyde:** 4% as diluted FORMALIN (37%)
18. **Glutaraldehyde:** 2%
19. **Boric acid:** 4% solution in warm water, 30% in Boroglycerine paint;
    BOROCIDE 10% oint, BOROSPIRIT 10% ear drops.
20. **Acetic acid:** 1–5%
21. **Silver nitrate:** 1%
22. **Zinc sulfate:** 1–4%; ZINCO-SULFA 0.1% eye drops, THIOSOL 2.5% lotion, THIOSOL FORTE 4% lotion.
23. **Gentian violet:** 0.5–1.0%
24. **Acriflavine:** 0.1–1%; ACRINOL 0.1% cream.
25. **Nitrofurazone:** 0.2–1.0%; FURACIN 0.2% cream, soluble oint, powder.

ECTOPARASITICIDES

1. **Permethrin:** *For scabies:* PERMITE, OMITE, NOMITE 5% cream; apply all over the body except face and head; wash after 8–12 hours; SCABERID 5% cream, 1% soap; SCABPER 5% lotion.
   For head lice: PERLICE, KERALICE 1% cream rinse, SCALTIX 1% lotion; massage about 30 g into the scalp, washoff after 10 min.
2. **Lindane (Gamma benzene hexachloride, BHC):**
   For pediculosis: apply to scalp and hair (taking care not to enter eyes), leave for 12–24 hr. (a shower cap may be used for long hair) and then wash off. If lice are still present repeat treatment after 1 week.
   For scabies: the lotion/cream is rubbed over the body (below neck) and a scrub bath taken 12–24 hr later. Single treatment suffices in most patients; can be repeated after a week;
   GAB 1% lotion, ointment; GAMADERM, SCABOMA 1% lotion; GAMASCAB 1% lotion, cream; ASCABIOL 1% emulsion with cetrimide 0.1%.
3. **Benzyl benzoate:** Apply 25% emulsion/ointment all over body (except face and neck) after a cleansing bath. Apply 2nd coat next day and wash off 24 hours later;
   DERMIN 25% lotion; SCABINDON 25% oint with DDT 1% and benzocaine 2%,
   BENZYLBENZOATE APPLICATION 25% lotion.
4. **Crotamiton:** Apply 10% lotion/cream twice at 24 hour interval and wash off the next day;
   CROTORAX 10% cream and lotion.
5. **Sulfur:** Apply 10% ointment daily for 3 days followed by soap-water bath on 4th day.
6. **Dicophane (DDT):** Apply 1–2% lotion/ointment all over except face, wash off next day;
   in SCABINDON 1% ointment with benzylbenzoate 25% and benzocaine 2%.
7. **Ivermectin:** 12 mg (0.2 mg/kg) oral single dose for scabies, head and body lice;
   IVERMECTOL, AVERTOL, IVERIN 3, 6 mg tabs, to be taken on empty stomach.

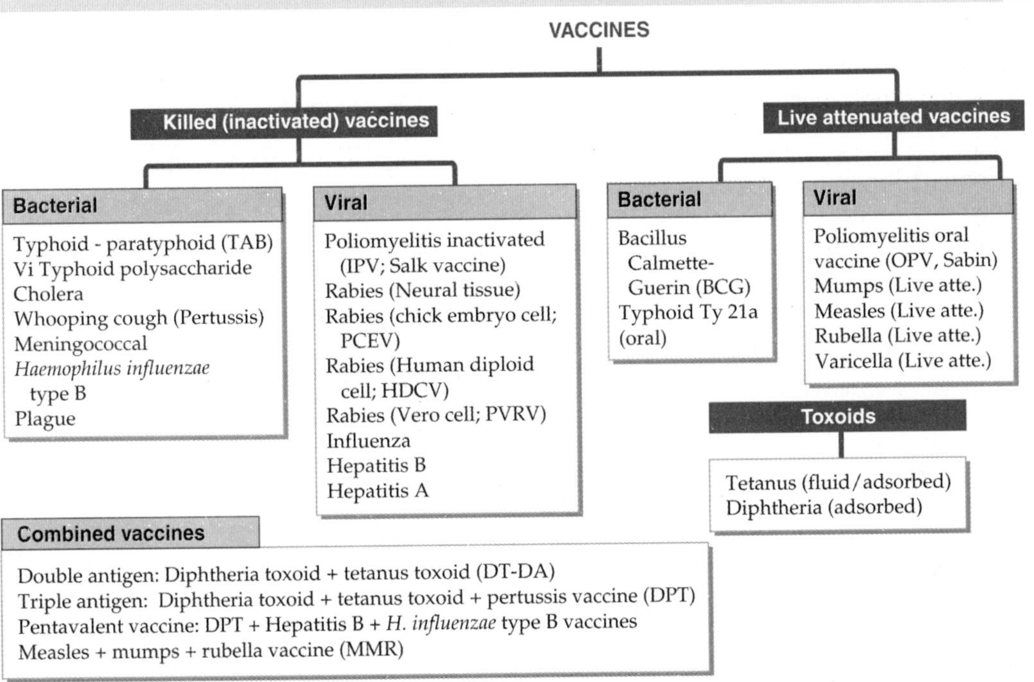
VACCINES
Killed (inactivated) vaccines
Live attenuated vaccines
Bacterial
Typhoid - paratyphoid (TAB)
Vi Typhoid polysaccharide
Cholera
Whooping cough (Pertussis)
Meningococcal
Haemophilus influenzae type B
Plague
Viral
Poliomyelitis inactivated (IPV; Salk vaccine)
Rabies (Neural tissue)
Rabies (chick embryo cell; PCEV)
Rabies (Human diploid cell; HDCV)
Rabies (Vero cell; PVRV)
Influenza
Hepatitis B
Hepatitis A
Bacterial
Bacillus Calmette-Guerin (BCG)
Typhoid Ty 21a (oral)
Viral
Poliomyelitis oral vaccine (OPV, Sabin)
Mumps (Live atte.)
Measles (Live atte.)
Rubella (Live atte.)
Varicella (Live atte.)
Toxoids
Tetanus (fluid/adsorbed)
Diphtheria (adsorbed)
Combined vaccines
Double antigen: Diphtheria toxoid + tetanus toxoid (DT-DA)
Triple antigen: Diphtheria toxoid + tetanus toxoid + pertussis vaccine (DPT)
Pentavalent vaccine: DPT + Hepatitis B + H. influenzae type B vaccines
Measles + mumps + rubella vaccine (MMR)

Preparations

1. Typhoid, Paratyphoid A, B (TAB vaccine): 0.5 ml s.c. 2–3 injections at 2–4 week intervals.
2. Vi Typhoid polysaccharide vaccine: 0.5 ml s.c./i.m. once, may be repeated after 3 years; VACTYPH, TYPHIM Vi, TYPHIVAX 0.025 mg in 0.5 ml inj.
3. Typhoid: Ty 21a oral vaccine: 3 caps taken in 3 doses on alternate days in-between meals; TYPHORAL *S. typhi* strain Ty21A 10^9 organism per cap.
4. Cholera vaccine: 0.5 ml s.c./i.m., repeat 1 ml after 4 weeks.
5. Whooping cough (pertussis) vaccine: 0.25–0.5 ml s.c./i.m. 3 doses at 4 week intervals in infants and children below 5 years age.
6. Meningococcal A & C vaccine: 0.5 ml s.c./i.m. single dose; MENINGOCOCCAL A & C, MENCEVAX A & C 0.5 ml amp, 5 ml vial.
7. Haemophilus influenzae type B (Hib) vaccine: 0.5 ml i.m. 2 doses at 8 weeks gap for children over 1 year, infants 2–12 month 3 doses; VAXEM HIB, HIB-TITER 0.5 ml and 5.0 ml vial.
8. Bacillus Calmette-Guérin (BCG) vaccine: 0.05 ml (neonate) 0.1 ml (older infants and children) intracutaneous injection in deltoid region.
9. Oral poliovirus vaccine (OPV, Sabin vaccine): 0.5 ml directly in the mouth at birth and at 6, 10, 14 weeks, booster dose at 15–18 month and at school entry.
10. Inactivated poliomyelitis vaccine (IPV, Salk vaccine):1 ml s.c. 3 injections at 4–6 week intervals and then 6–12 months later, booster doses every 5 years.
11. Purified chick embryo cell vaccine (PCEV): 2.5 IU/ml inj; 0.1 ml intradermal (i.d.) over deltoid of both arms on days 0, 3, 7 and over one arm only on days 28 and 90 (total 8 injections) for post exposure prophylaxis of rabies; for primary prophylaxis 3 doses of 0.1 ml i.d. on days 0, 7 and 28; RABIPUR 1 ml inj.

12. **Human diploid cell vaccine (HDCV):** 2.5 i.u./ml inj; 0.2 ml i.d. over both deltoids on days 0, 3 and 7 and over one only on days 28 and 90 (total 8 injections), for post exposure prophylaxis of rabies; for primary prophylaxis 3 doses of 0.1 ml each i.d. on days 0, 7 and 28; MERIEUX HDC 2.5 IU inj.
13. **Purified vero cell rabies vaccine (PVRV):** 2.5 i.u./ml inj; 0.2 ml i.d. over both deltoids on days 0, 3 and 7 and over one only on days 28 and 90 (total 8 injections) for post exposure prophylaxis of rabies; for primary prophylaxis 3 doses of 0.1 ml each i.d. on days 0, 7 and 28; VERORAB 1 ml inj; VEROVAX-R 0.5 ml inj.
14. **Influenza virus vaccine:** 0.25 ml (6 month–3 year age), 0.5 ml (> 3 year age) i.m. 2 injections 1–2 months apart; VAXIGRIP 0.5 ml prefilled syringe.
15. **Hepatitis B vaccine:** 1 ml i.m. in deltoid muscle at 0, 1, 6 months (children < 10 yr 0.5 ml injection in the thigh); ENGERIX-B, ENIVAC-HB 1 ml (single dose) and 10 ml (multiple dose) vials.
16. **Hepatitis A vaccine:** 0.5 ml i.m. single dose, may be repeated after 6 months; AVAXIM 0.5 ml prefilled syringe, HAVRIX 0.5 ml, 1.0 ml inj.
17. **Measles vaccine live attenuated:** 1000 $TCID_{50}$ s.c. single dose; ROUVAX, RIMEVAX, M-VAC 1000 $TCID_{50}$/vial inj.
18. **Rubella vaccine:** 1000 $TCID_{50}$ i.m./s.c. single dose; R-VAC 1000 $TCID_{50}$ in 0.5 ml inj.
19. **Measles-Mumps-Rubella (MMR) vaccine:** 0.5 ml i.m./deep s.c. single dose; TRIMOVAX lyophilized measles 1000 $TCID_{50}$ of Schwarz strain, mumps 5000 $TCID_{50}$ and rubella 1000 $TCID_{50}$ per unit dose (0.5 ml) vial. TRESIVAC lyophilized measles 5000 $TCID_{50}$ of Edmonston Zagreb strain, mumps 5000 $TCID_{50}$ and rubella 4000 $TCID_{50}$ per unit dose (0.5 ml) vial.
20. **Varicella vaccine:** 0.5 ml s.c. single dose for children 1–12 years, and 2 doses 6–10 weeks apart in those >12 years. VARILRIX, OKAVAX 0.5 ml inj.
21. **Tetanus toxoid:** 0.5 ml i.m. (also s.c.) 2 doses 4–6 weeks apart for primary immunization, booster dose every 10 years, or after a risky wound; TETANUS TOXOID ADSORBED 0.5 ml amp, 5.0 ml vial.

22. **Diphtheria toxoid:** 0.5 ml i.m. 2–3 injections 4–6 weeks apart in children below 6 years, booster doses after 1 year and at school entry.
23. **Double antigen (Diphtheria-Tetanus toxoids):** 0.5 ml i.m. 2–3 injections 4–8 weeks apart; DUAL ANTIGEN 0.5 ml amp, 5 ml vial.
24. **Triple antigen (Diphtheria-Pertussis-Tetanus, DPT):** 0.5 ml i.m. 2–3 injections 4–8 weeks apart between 3–9 months age, booster dose at 18 months age; TRIPVAC 0.5 ml amp, 10 ml multidose vial.

ANTISERA AND IMMUNE GLOBULINS

Antisera (from Horse)

Tetanus antitoxin (ATS)
Gas gangrene antitoxin (AGS)
Diphtheria antitoxin (ADS)
Antirabies serum (ARS)
Antisnake venom polyvalent

Immune globulins (Human)

Normal human gamma globulin
Rho(D) immune globulin
Tetanus immune globulin
Rabies immune globulin
Hepatitis-B immune globulin

Preparations

1. **Tetanus antitoxin (ATS):** Prophylactic 1500–3000 IU, i.m. or s.c.; therapeutic 50,000–100,000 IU part i.v. and rest i.m.;
   TETANUS ANTITOXIN 750 IU, 1500 IU, 5000 IU, 10,000 IU, 20,000 IU, and 50,000 IU in 1–10 ml ampoules.
   TETANUS IMMUNE SERUM (enzyme refined, equine) 10,000 and 20,000 IU vials.
2. **Gasgangrene antitoxin (AGS):** Prophylactic 10,000 IU; therapeutic 30,000–75,000 IU s.c./i.m./i.v.; AGGS 10,000 IU amp.

3. **Diphtheria antitoxin (ADS):** 20,000–40,000 IU i.m. or i.v. for pharyngeal/laryngeal disease of upto 48 hour duration. Higher dose (upto 100,000 IU may be needed).
   DIPHTHERIA ANTITOXIN 10,000 IU in 10 ml amp.
4. **Antirabies serum (ARS):** 40 IU/kg infiltrated round the bite wound; IMORAB 1000 IU/5 ml inj.
5. **Antisnake venom polyvalent:** 20 ml i.v. repeated 1–6 hourly till symptoms of envenomation disappear (total upto 300 ml); ANTISNAKE VENOM SERUM POLYVALENT, ASVS lyophilized vial to be reconstituted with 10 ml distilled water; each ml of reconstituted serum neutralizes 0.6 mg cobra, 0.6 mg Russel's viper, 0.45 mg of saw scaled viper and 0.45 mg of Krait venoms.
6. **Normal human gamma globulin:** 0.02–1.0 ml/kg i.m.; GAMMALIN, GLOBUNAL, Sii GAMMA GLOBULIN, GAMAFINE 10%, 16.5% injection in 1, 2 ml amps; for i.v. use sii IVGG, ZY-IVGG 0.1–0.4 g/kg/day; 0.5, 1.0, 2.5 g vials.
7. **Rho(D) immune globulin:** (*See* p. 177)
8. **Tetanus immune globulin:** Prophylactic 250–500 IU, therapeutic 3000–6000 IU i.m. and/or 250–500 IU intrathecal; Sii TIG 250 IU (liquid), 500 IU (lyophilized), TETNAL 250 IU/2 ml inj., TETAGAM 250 IU/ml inj.
9. **Rabies immune globulin (HRIG):** 20 IU/kg infiltrated round the bite on the day of exposure, excess injected i.m.; BERIRAB-P 300 IU/2 ml and 750 IU/5 ml inj; RABGLOB 300 IU/2 ml inj.
10. **Hepatitis B immune globulin:** 1000–2000 IU (adults), 32–48 IU/kg (children) to be administered within 7 days of exposure; HEPAGLOB 100 IU (0.5 ml) 200 IU (1 ml) per vial for i.m. inj.

Index of Nonproprietary Names of Drugs

A

B

C

D

E

F

M

Q

R

T

Index of Proprietary (Brand) Names of Drugs

B

C

D

F

G

H

M

N

O

Q

R

S

T

U

Z